FOREWORD

Radiant health and optimal wellness does not occur by accident.

When I first met Dori Luneski, I was immediately struck by her vibrant and youthful appearance. Here was a lady who admitted to being just shy of her 65th birthday and yet had the appearance and energy of someone at least 20 years younger. After sharing with me the story of her own dramatic health transformation, I realized that I had found that "rarest of birds"...a health practitioner who demonstrated unequivocally that she knew and lived the natural laws of wellness that most of us are either largely ignorant of or only give lip service to.

Times have changed. Due to the failure of modern allopathic medicine to stem the tide of the epidemic of chronic disease and premature death in this country, there is at long last a heightened awareness of the need for personal responsibility. The importance of making nutritional and other lifestyle choices that promote wellness rather than "disease" is finally settling into the consciousness of the masses. Simultaneously, there is an increasing need for health care providers and healers from various alternative disciplines to demonstrate the highest level of competence, clarity, and compassion in assisting those whom we are called upon to serve. And that is as it should be.

Nature dictates that true wellness is multi-dimensional and encompasses every aspect of who we are...spiritually, mentally, emotionally, and physically. No part of the equation can be ignored without sacrificing some level of benefit. But how does one sort through all the hype and commercialism to find a personal road map to that elusive destination called "wellness?" The ever-increasing panorama of choices in the many diverse disciplines loosely termed alternative health or complimentary medicine is at best confusing, even to those who have taken on the task of educating themselves to the many options.

For example, nutrition is perhaps the single most important component of a sound program for wellness. Yet even in this one category there is an overwhelming amount of information and advice being given…much of it confusing and contradictory. Just what is a "good" diet anyway, and is it the same for everyone? What supplements should I take and how many? How do I even know if these supplements are doing me any good? What about herbs and homeopathics? How much can I do on my own as opposed to going to "experts" who may or may not have my best interests at heart?

The "psychology of wellness" is an equally diverse and uncharted course. How much does the inner-directed activity of positive thinking, creative imagery, mirroring, and attitudinal change really impact on how we feel, both physically and emotionally? Can I really "re-invent" myself using mind-power alone?

The dilemma is obvious. In the midst of an unprecedented explosion of information and increasingly abundant choices for charting our course toward wellness, the need for simple, sound, and user-friendly advice is at an all-time premium.

In her latest book, The Power to Heal, Dori Luneski presents a program for optimal health that is not only based on sound scientific principles but is also imminently practical. She doesn't just "talk the talk" of someone with a wealth of book knowledge and little or no real world experience. She is, above all, a true example of someone who has "walked the walk" by going through her own metamorphosis from a bedridden patient with debilitating disease who had been essentially written off by traditional allopathic medicine, to one of the most vibrantly healthy people I have ever met.

And beyond that, through her writing, lecturing, and clinical practice, Dori is educating, coaching, and inspiring thousands of others to go through similar health transformations. I count myself among those who have been privileged to tap into her well-spring of knowledge and insight that truly sets her apart from the rank and file of practitioners, who may talk about promoting health but largely only provide symptomatic management of disease.

You hold in your hands a priceless resource of sound practical advice and time honored wisdom that can lead you to

THE POWER TO HEAL

ON ALL LEVELS:

SPIRITUAL
MENTAL
EMOTIONAL
PHYSICAL

By

Dori Luneski, R.N., N.D.

FOREWARD BY Matthew Silver, M.D.

1stBooks - rev. 7/25/02

ACKNOWLEDGMENTS

To...

Marijane Thompson, whose excellence in everything she does makes my hard days easier. Without her valuable assistance, the completion of this book would have been immeasurably more difficult.

To...

my spiritual leaders, who strengthened my awareness that I am God's child and He has a plan for me.

To...

My husband, Eddie, who calms as well as energizes my life, and is an example of not just having spiritual beliefs, but living by them.

To...

Rebecca Grace Jones, for her artistic drawings.

I DEDICATE THIS BOOK

TO MY HUSBAND, EDDIE DON ARCHULETA

I HAVE NEVER BEEN RICH BEFORE,
BUT YOU HAVE POURED
INTO MY HEART'S DOOR
A GOLDEN HOARD.

MY WEALTH IS THE VISION SHARED,
THE SAMENESS OF FEELING,
THE FEAST OF THE SOUL PREPARED
BY YOU FOR ME.

TOGETHER WE WANDER THROUGH
THE WOODED WAYS.
REMEMBERING OLD WHILE NEW IS
SEEN THROUGH OUR GAZE.

I LOOK FOR NO GREATER PRIZE
THAN YOUR SOFT VOICE.
THE STEADINESS OF YOUR EYES
IS MY HEART'S CHOICE.

I HAVE NEVER BEEN RICH BEFORE,
BUT I DIVINE
YOUR STEP ON MY SUNLIT FLOOR,
AND WEALTH IS MINE!

TABLE OF CONTENTS

CHAPTER 3

CHAPTER 4

CHAPTER 5

CHAPTER 6

levels of enhanced well-being far exceeding what most of us have come to accept as "normal." Use it well.

Matthew Silver, M.D.

Wellness Educator and Lead Physician Marketing Executive for FreeLife International

DISCLAIMER

THE POWER TO HEAL is not intended to treat disease, in any way interfere with diagnostic procedures or treatment by any medical practitioner, or be construed as medical advice. This book may seem controversial to some; it is not intended to satisfy modern science. The opinions herein are strictly those of the author. The "first do no harm" recommendations in this book are meant to be guidelines to assist the body to work at optimal performance, or heal itself if possible. Even in the face of serious illness, the principles of wellness should not be ignored. The author urges anyone having a health concern to see a licensed practitioner for evaluation. The application of any concepts in this book without the consent of a licensed practitioner is not encouraged; however, it is your constitutional right to decide how you wish to treat your body. The author and the publisher assume no liability for the implementation of any material presented.

WHY YOU SHOULD READ THIS BOOK

This book is for those who are "sick and tired of being sick and tired." It is for those who seek help and are told that their physical examination and blood chemistry is normal, and are left with unanswered questions as to why they feel so ill. This book is for those who are pacified with a drug, because that is what the doctor thinks is expected. The patient is told to come back if symptoms do not improve; by then health may have deteriorated to the point where other medication and/or surgery is recommended.

This book is for those who have been told to eat a "well-balanced diet," but are given minimum information about the laws of wellness. They are left to the mercy of the food industry propaganda. The handouts from medical organizations for dietary advice have such surface information, they only add to the frustration and confusion when nothing seems to help.

This book is for those who have learned that the health-care industry has little to offer for "chronic poor health" except a quick prescription, a pat on the back with no help for your symptoms, or a referral to another doctor with similar disappointing results. A barrage of expensive tests can seem unnecessary; some can have inaccurate information; some tests can be dangerous, with serious side effects or reactions.

If you had a pain in your side today for the first time, and a week from now a doctor diagnosed colon cancer, you did not know *yesterday* you had colon cancer. It can take five to twenty years for the body to degenerate to the degree you experience a symptom. That symptom was a sign body degeneration had reach a stage in which the body could no longer suppress what was developing. This book is for those people who want to assume responsibility for their "wellness," and have a better change of controlling the development of disease.

There are many people looking for a practical, reasonable method of taking responsibility for their health. This book will provide guidance through the confusion that discourages so many people, who are trying to nurture themselves and their families in a sick world.

Treating disease is complicated; preventing disease is simple. This book simplifies a subject that has been made complicated by modern medicine's treatment of disease, and made confusing by the abundance of preventive medicine's options.

It is true that medically trained people can best treat you for traumatic or acute illnesses. When I broke my hip skiing, I did not ask for a cup of herb tea. However, Robert Mendelsohn, M.D. says in his book *CONFESSIONS OF A MEDICAL HERETIC*:

"I BELIEVE THAT, DESPITE ALL THE SUPER TECHNOLOGY AND ELITE BEDSIDE MANNER THAT'S SUPPOSED TO MAKE YOU FEEL ABOUT AS WELL CARED FOR AS AN ASTRONAUT ON THE WAY TO THE MOON, THE GREATEST DANGER TO YOUR HEALTH IS THE DOCTOR WHO PRACTICES MODERN MEDICINE."

No one is as interested in your health as you are. You alone suffer pain, loss of life enjoyment, premature aging, and untimely death. You go to a modern doctor to feel better *NOW;* too often that is all you get. But, having a symptom relieved is not health. The name of the symptom, the name of the disease is NOT YOUR PROBLEM! Your problem is what *CAUSED* the symptom or disease.

You can read *dozens* of separate books, building knowledge on different health subjects. Too often people do not read enough different health topics to put together a complete wellness program that works *"holistically"* in the body. My book gives you ALL THE BASIC LAWS OF HEALTH in *one* book, so you do not miss important health considerations. **This is YOUR life** ... you must assume responsibility for *preventing* disease.

My own 20 year illness, added to the trials, struggles, setbacks and successes for another 20 years, have enabled me to organize this very practical approach for you, the "health student." The "laws" of wellness will help you to care for yourself and your loved ones. The result will be the enthusiasm that helps you make healthier daily choices. The payoff for making better decisions is doing the things you really want ... feeling good ... and enjoying life to the fullest.

To my active nursing license, I added four years as a rehabilitation specialist, twelve years working with holistic practitioners, and six years as a psychiatric nurse. I then obtained my diploma in Doctor of Naturopathy from the Clayton School of Natural Healing in Birmingham, Alabama. Twenty years of holistic research has culminated into this presentation.

My first book, FOUNTAIN OF HEALTH AND FITNESS is out of print. My second book, HEALTH METAMORPHOSIS was edited and reprinted for the second edition. To you dear reader ... I give you the best of all my accumulated knowledge in THE POWER TO HEAL.

Deciding on the title of this book was a spiritual experience. For weeks I lived with word association, hoping to find a title that would entice people to take a second look. Even the best books can be easily lost in the book jungle. I asked God to help me find the right words for a title. My friend invited me to attend the Naval Academy Chapel Sunday service in Annapolis. At the beginning of the service I had an overpowering feeling that the name of the book was in the program. I did not listen to the service at all, but concentrated on the program to locate this sign. Many words triggered my interest, but after putting words together in my mind, nothing seemed right. I did not stop scanning the print, because the strong feeling continued that "the name of the book was in the program." Then I saw in a sentence the words ... power to heal. I immediately was overwhelmed with a feeling of warmth. Tears came to my eyes. A sense of peace enveloped my body. I knew the name of the book was THE POWER TO HEAL. God has guided me for years, and now ... dear reader ... I give you my best.

Enjoy ...

Dori Luneski, R.N., N.D.
Naturopathic Practitioner

INTRODUCTION

Metamorphosis is a change. A slow, wriggling caterpillar pupates; for a time the gray pupa hangs from a twig, while within, a miracle is taking place. The pupa at last splits open, and the butterfly is born, to greet the flowers with beautiful rainbow wings. A human can undergo metamorphosis, too. The cocoon of a sickly body can be broken open, and the healthy, vital new person can escape.

In my life I have undergone a metamorphosis; now people marvel at my excellent health. I was so crippled I could barely function; today at 68, I am vital, full of energy, and feel terrific! People who knew me when I was ill are amazed at my improved health. People meeting me for the first time are impressed with my youthful appearance and vitality. I was fortunate enough to find a constructive path to better health that treated the *CAUSE* of my illness, not just the symptoms. Whether you are ill and want to feel better, or just want to protect your current health, you do not have to search for years, as I did. If you follow THE "LAWS" OF WELLNESS in this book, metamorphosis can happen to you!

Modern medical technology has made it possible for many people to live longer lives. Living a long life, however, should not be your only goal. You should want to be healthy, active, productive and enthusiastic for life in your senior years. The definition of health in Webster's dictionary states: "Physical and mental well-being, soundness, freedom from defeat, pain or disease, normality of mental and physical function." The next line was what I was looking for in the definition, "Health is something different from strength. It is universal good condition." Just because you were able to get up this morning does not imply any degree of health! Health is achieved only when you have FREEDOM from symptoms on all levels ... spiritual, mental, emotional, and physical.

In this book we will examine self-health; how you can practice principles of health that allow your body to work at optimum performance, or heal itself if there is not irreversible damage. Modern medicine practitioners best understand the complexities of the human body, but everyone should have a basic understanding of how to make choices for his or her well being. *THE POWER TO HEAL* will teach you how what you eat, think, and do affects your health.

[] [] [] [] [] []

My path to good health has been a long one. I realize now that the harm I was doing to my body did not immediately make me sick, and the good health practices I later learned did not cure me in a week. With such a slow process, you do not see immediate results from any action, whether health building or health destroying. What started as a few annoying symptoms took years to develop into debilitating illness.

My first symptom at age 25 was pain in my ribs. I did not realize it at the time, but that was the beginning of gradually deteriorating health that left me nearly an invalid 20 years later. It started when a doctor treated my symptoms with an anti-inflammatory drug. When I moved to Eugene, Oregon, a doctor continued my treatment for the same unresolved distress. For four years, I was treated with a variety of medications. Each symptom was treated separately; I was referred to specialists, each of whom was involved in only a narrow field of medicine. None of these physicians suggested looking for the *CAUSE* of my complaints. Some medications did help suppress the symptoms, but I never felt *well*.

As my health deteriorated, I developed a disease one of my doctors called Polymyositis (an inflammatory muscle disease that is a branch of Lupus). This diagnosis was not the beginning of new hope; in fact, I was about to embark on a 12-year nightmare. In the first year, my doctors prescribed so many drugs that charts were necessary to keep it all straight. Some medications produced side effects; other medications were required to counteract the side effects. In some cases still other medications were prescribed to counteract the side effects of those medications.

Our society has learned to accept the end result of poor health and not ask doctors to explain what *CAUSED* their illness. In many cases the doctors may not even know. My doctors quickly discouraged my questions. They did not encourage me to take part in decisions concerning my health. They wanted me to "trust them." Symptoms were treated, but causes were ignored.

My doctors *NEVER* recommended supplements. I was told by one doctor after another, "Just eat a good diet." I ate what is generally regarded as a "good diet." Based on our society's standards, that meant low fiber, too little raw food, too much cooked and processed food, excess of mucous forming and poorly digested red meat and dairy products, high fat, refined sugar, junk food, and food additives. None of the doctors discussed the details of what a *health building* diet should be. I am a Registered Nurse, but even in the nursing program, the laws of wellness discussed in this book were not emphasized.

As a nurse, I had been taught to follow directions. I was taught to trust what the doctors said was correct. I was cared for with modern technology's finest equipment, and medical specialists using continuous drug therapy and multiple surgeries. Despite that, I became a medical disaster by the time I was 45. At one time or another, I suffered all of these symptoms:

Overweight
Unhealthy nails, hair, and skin
Chronic fatigue
Pain in every joint; weak, painful muscles
Severe constipation
Backaches, headaches, and debilitating neck pain
Cold body and extremities all year
Chronic vaginal yeast infections
Sexual desire completely void
PMS and painful periods
Extreme emotional highs and lows; anxiety attacks
Chronic tension and irritability
Frequent colds that could last months
Kidney pain and one kidney stone
Acute gallbladder attack

Sore, burning mouth; frequent mouth sores
Problem getting to sleep and staying asleep
Chest pain; very rapid pulse; sore ribs
Stomach pain and nausea after meals
Sleepy after meals; gas and bloating

Doctors never treated my whole body; they merely treated each symptom with drugs or surgery. Eventually I developed intolerance to most of the drugs they prescribed. My doctors started thinking of me as a hypochondriac, because I still had so many symptoms when some of their tests showed what they considered to be normal results. They had no explanation for my lack of progress, so they said I was "stressed out," and recommended psychiatric counseling. Years of therapy did not improve my general health at all. The only change was an increase in symptoms from the variety of drugs they prescribed for me.

A friend informed me about another kind of doctor who treated food allergies. Since I had been told everything that could be done was being done, a new doctor did not seem necessary. I was tired of the frustration and disappointment every time I sought a new physician. When I finally agreed to see this new doctor, my life changed dramatically!

Fuller Royal, M.D. approached my problems from a different point of view. His concern about the CAUSE of my symptoms was a refreshing change from just treating the symptoms. Dr. Royal concluded my problems to be both food allergies and chemical sensitivities. I was hospitalized in a chemically controlled environment under the care of Joseph Morgan, M.D. After a total water fast, I was tested with food not grown with chemical fertilizer or sprayed with any chemical. In two weeks, I learned more about what was actually CAUSING my many symptoms than my other doctors had determined in 20 years. Some of the symptoms explained by food and chemical testing were:

Beef made me depressed and tearful.
Milk gave me joint pains.

Corn made my muscles hurt.

Soy made my legs ache.

Gluten (wheat, oats, rye, barley, possibly buckwheat) caused rib, chest and stomach pain.

Chemicals in my clothing and environment caused headaches, fatigue, depression, irritability, and neck pain.

My medical mismanagement left many scars, but none more difficult to deal with than chemical sensitivities. Since World War II, we have become a chemically oriented society. Locating chemical-free food, natural fiber clothing, natural household furnishings, and non-chemical supplies was not easy or inexpensive. Solving my problems quickly was critical. My family was often shocked, frustrated, and angry at how complicated our lives had become.

I was angry with the medical profession for the way they treated me, and resented the loss of enjoyable years, and aggravation to my family. After years of believing medical science would cure me, the final realization that I was responsible for my own health was difficult to accept. Making daily choices to heal my body, and protect my health, was a new way of life.

After a year and a half, I was well enough to work in a holistic health clinic, and organized seminars to share the health techniques I had learned. I took personal growth seminars, and started teaching classes on positive thinking and stress management. I learned there was more to health than improved diet, and avoidance of substances that made me ill. I learned *balanced* health was on all levels of spiritual, mental, emotional, and physical.

[] [] [] [] [] []

THE POWER TO HEAL is dedicated to assisting you in making choices for your best health interest, now and in the future. Health is simple … it is disease that is so complicated. **If you practice the principles of the basic "laws" of wellness,**

your body can take better care of itself on all levels of spiritual, mental, emotional, and physical.

Your journey to better health could be likened to you taking a walk on a winding trail. Your path may turn gradually or have some sharp curves. It may stray occasionally from the main course. With a challenging stream to cross, you may have to control your fear as you balance across a fallen log. You may need to stop and rest. You may wonder how you can go on, but when at last you reach the beautiful view from the summit, you realize it was well worth it.

I want my story to give you new hope. If you are one of the many people who have struggled vainly with modern medicine, you need this book desperately. Application of the information in the next six chapters can perform miracles. It took many years of researching the *bottom line* causes of illness and disease to uncover important details in the search for wellness. Information on Leaky Gut Syndrome causing digestive and intestinal symptoms, and Wilson's Syndrome dealing with metabolism, must be evaluated as part of the whole health picture. Your health could depend on you understanding the energy loss from normal body function due to electromagnetic polluted frequencies in our "new and improved" world. Too many people struggling with physical symptoms do not understand mental and emotional relationship to physical stress. This ignored information in favor of just treating the symptoms, may produce unrewarding results. I am proud to present this text in such a complete format.

I no longer am willing to blindly follow medical recommendations that only treat the symptoms in chronic illness. I would however, seek medical evaluation if following the "LAWS" OF WELLNESS did not produce positive results in a reasonable period of time. Our societies health care program would benefit greatly by everyone working together, with the best of both preventive medicine and modern medicine. Our current health care system is not health care, but mostly disease care.

Right now is the perfect time for you to start on your path to health metamorphosis! As you consider each new idea, remember you are not going through this alone. Let us turn the page together. I will help you learn the principles that allow your body to work at optimum performance, or heal itself.

This is your health journey ...

enjoy it!!!

CHAPTER 1

POSITIVE THINKING
IS POSSIBILITY THINKING

Sometimes life IS rough. Positive thinking does not guarantee you anything; however, negative thinking GUARANTEES it will be harder to deal with your problems. Positive thinking is POSSIBILITY THINKING ... and that comes from the loving acceptance of yourself. With positive thinking you are OPEN to the options that can make a difference, because you WANT TO ENJOY LIFE. You can make that hard ... or ... you can make it easy. It's your choice!

This poem from *HOW TO SURVIVE THE LOSS OF A LOVE* written by Colgrove, Bloomfield, and McWilliams, radiates with positive imagery:

> **The world is good.**
> **I feel whole and directed.**
> **Touch my Joy with me.**
> **I cannot keep**
> **my smiles**
> **in single file.**

THE GREATEST CAUSE OF ILLNESS IS NEGATIVE EMOTIONS. You may believe that continuous stress caused you to develop negative emotions. You may believe you cannot change much in your life because you cannot get rid of your stress. You may not be able to change the negative events in your life, but you can learn to control your ATTITUDE towards them. *This is one of my favorite quotes about attitude:*

> *The longer I live, the more I realize the impact of attitude on life. Attitude, to me, is more important than facts. It is more important than the past, than education, than money, than circumstances, than failures, than successes,*

1

than what other people think or say or do. It will make or break a company, a church, a home. The remarkable thing is, we have a choice every day regarding the attitude we embrace for that day. We cannot change the inevitable. The only thing we can do is play the one string we have, and that is our attitude. I am convinced life is 10 percent what happens to me, and 90 percent how I react to it. An so it is with you; we are in charge of our attitudes.

- Charles Swindoll

How you think and feel is based a lot on your self-esteem, and affects everything you do ... every relationship, every task, every choice, every second of your day! The *character* you develop is from your *attitude* about your lifetime of trials, errors, and daily struggles that bring out the best in you. CHARACTER BUILDS SELF-ESTEEM.

The will to self-love is the deepest of all desires. You are involved with the greatest adventure of your life ... to improve your self-esteem, to create more meaning in your life, and in the lives of others. Creating a better self-image does not create new abilities, but it does release the ones you already have.

"LIFE'S GREATEST ACHIEVEMENT IS THE CONTINUAL REMAKING OF YOURSELF SO THAT AT LAST YOU KNOW HOW TO LIVE."

- Norman Vincent Peale

ENTHUSIASM FOR LIFE IS THE MOST IMPORTANT PREDICTOR OF WELLNESS. It is impossible to attain good health without a positive attitude towards life. This is why POSITIVE THINKING is the first chapter of this book. The best diet and exercise program in the world will not provide the health you expect, if you do not approach each day and each task with enthusiasm.

"FINISH EVERY DAY AND BE DONE WITH IT. YOU HAVE DONE WHAT YOU COULD. SOME BLUNDERS AND ABSURDITIES NO DOUBT CREPT IN; FORGET THEM AS SOON AS YOU CAN. TOMORROW IS A NEW DAY; BEGIN IT WELL AND SERENELY. THIS DAY IS ALL THAT IS GOOD AND FAIR. IT IS TOO DEAR, WITH ITS HOPES AND INVITATIONS, TO WASTE A MOMENT ON THE YESTERDAYS."

- Ralph Waldo Emerson

Most people, at one time or another, transfer their energy in negative directions ... towards conflict, stagnation, and isolation. To be healthy, you must learn to channel your energy in a direction that will build health. Wisdom is knowing what to do next! Wisdom lies in the ability to forgive ourselves and others of human failings; and when we tumble, pick ourselves up and learn from the experience. Today you are learning to do it better tomorrow. That is what life is all about ... to become stronger (not weaker) from your experiences.

[] [] [] [] [] []

IT ALL STARTS WITH POSITIVE ENERGY. That increases your ENTHUSIASM so you *want to participate in life*, not just observe it. If you dread Saturday night, Sundays are no fun, and holidays are even worse, you need to take a good look at YOURSELF. A person who CHOOSES to be lonely any day can also CHOOSE not to ... any day! Do not allow television to fill all your time. It should be used for information or relaxation, but not for a way to escape from life. *The following are ways to GET INTO ACTION:*

* **Take personal development seminars or lectures, read personal growth books, listen to personal growth tapes and videos, or watch stimulating television programs.** They assist in bringing out the

3

giant that is inside you. *Consider these options with contact information in Resource References:*

1. Robert H. Schuller, Hour of Power TV Ministries, *specializing* in transforming personal lives.

2. Joyce Meyer TV Ministries provides *powerful* guidance for personal development.

3. Ed Young, The Winning Walk TV Ministries provides *inspiring* spiritual guidance.

4. James Kennedy, Coral Ridge TV Ministries, provides *insightful* spiritual growth.

5. Arthur Caliandro, home church replacement for Norman Vincent Peale.

6. Joel Osteen, insightful spiritual guidance.

7. Check calendar events of local newspapers.

* **Connect with your Creator** and let the light that shines *within* provide the enthusiasm that will be your driving force. Allow your intuition, or vibes to direct your energy into becoming all that you can be.

> *... that you will be filled with His mighty, glorious strength so that you can keep going no matter what happens ...*
>
> Colossians 1:11

This is part of a call to worship at a church service:

> By your powerful Spirit,
> turn our fear to courage
> and our confusion to confidence.

Ask yourself, *"How is it between me and the Lord?"* Find the time to look within yourself ... stop ... reflect ... then asked yourself again, *"How is it between me and the Lord?"* You may experience the strength and guidance you need, if you took the time to connect.

* **Take an adult education class or other educational opportunity** through a university, community college, or city parks department. I took flower identification, bird watching, and animal tracking classes to enrich my hikes. Learning through classes will expand your horizons, and reward you both in knowledge and social enjoyment. TO SEARCH IS TO NEVER EXPERIENCE BOREDOM!

* **Experience creativity** by DOING what you want to do, not just thinking about it. The only thing that stops the creative person inside you, is your negative subconscious *that you put there.*

> *A friend admired my oil paintings and said she had always wanted to paint. She denied her ability. When I finally persuaded her to paint with me, she completed a beautiful mountain scene. She displays her work with* **pride, and accepts compliments with a big smile.**

All the poems I have written in my life have been at the height of feeling good about myself. Poetry is an effective balancing mechanism because it is both left brain logical, and right brain creative. Thus, it can balance the cerebral hemispheres and reduce tension.

"INSTEAD OF ONE ASPIRIN, TAKE TWO POEMS."

> - psychiatrist Dr. Jack Leedy's advice when his patients have trouble sleeping.

5

* **Get involved in fun activities** because life does not always have to be a struggle. Play may be the most vital thing you do, because it will renew you. If you cannot enjoy a good time, and you feel like a victim, you may be coming from the belief system that you cannot be happy, and life is hard. Through your negative thoughts and choices you will make sure life stays hard, because it confirms your belief system. Play balances the cerebral hemispheres, so you are not all left-brain thinking. Imbalance in the cerebral hemispheres can stress the immune system.

When you are having fun, you also need to learn the art of relaxation. Unfortunately, many people try to relax at the same pace that they lead the rest of their lives. *True relaxation is becoming sensitive to one's basic needs for self-awareness, and thoughtful reflection.* Many people are so pressure oriented they do not take time to satisfy their own basic needs (discussed in more detail on page 44). *Not satisfying your basic needs is an almost guaranteed program for illness.* Our production-oriented society is so task directed that even vacations become whirlwind projects. When some people return home after a vacation, they are still exhausted.

"REST IS ACTION WITHOUT FRICTION."

- Robert H. Schuller

Remember RELAXATION, and not achievement is your main goal. *Two important rules in deciding what activity to pick are:*

1. Do not be afraid to try something new and different.

2. Choose the activity YOU enjoy, not always what other people want you to do.

* **Laughing** gives the body a mini-workout, as it involves virtually every major body system. For millions of people life is like a toothache with no money to see a dentist. They finally give up and accept the pain with all the elements of being a victim. They struggle for survival using negative manipulation, and are shocked when life gets worse. *They lose a valuable link to survival ... humor!*

[] [] [] [] [] []

HOW TO RESOLVE A PROBLEM

We cannot laugh all day if there are real problems. To resolve a problem, you need a plan. *Always remember that ACTION is the antidote for worry.* Have a separate piece of paper for each problem, and answer the following questions **on each problem.** *Then prioritize them in order of urgency, and decide on a place to start!*

- WHAT IS THE *REAL* PROBLEM?

Many people worry before they get all the facts. Deal only with the facts! A situation handled with *all the facts correct,* could keep a problem from getting out of hand.

- WHAT IS THE *CAUSE* OF THE PROBLEM?

This should give you some hints on how to deal with it. Remember to assume responsibility for any part you play in the problem. This is a time for *self-assessment and honesty!*

- WHAT ARE *ALL* THE POSSIBLE SOLUTIONS?

No one can know all the uncertainties, but you can give an educated guess to the solutions based on the known facts. *This is the time to think, and not be emotional.* Future "what-ifs" and past "if-onlys" can only drive you crazy with speculation. It keeps you in a negative attitude that prevents you from forming a GAME PLAN *to resolve the issue.*

- PICK A POSSIBLE SOLUTION AND *ACT* ON IT!

WORRY IS DEFINITELY NOT ACTION! Worry is a negative thought that wastes energy ... and that can prevent you from solving the problem. One of the biggest causes of chronic worry is low self-esteem. However, when you worry with a positive mental attitude, it can be to your advantage, and lead to solutions.

DEAL WITH THE FACTS ...
ACT ON THE FACTS ...
DO THE BEST YOU CAN TODAY ... BECAUSE TODAY IS THE TOMORROW YOU WORRIED ABOUT YESTERDAY!

"WE SHALL HAVE NO BETTER CONDITIONS IN THE FUTURE IF WE ARE SATISFIED WITH ALL THOSE WHICH WE HAVE AT PRESENT."

- Thomas Edison

EXAMINE YOUR SELF-ESTEEM

Reorganize priorities because you deserve a part of each day for yourself. If you are swamped with tasks you do not feel like doing, or responsibilities not of your own choosing, perhaps it is time to reorganize your priorities. You should examine your self-esteem, if you believe your life is not under your control.

Your self-esteem may not always be from conscious thoughts, but may be from your subconscious. Your subconscious is the source of information for your conscious mind, and stores all the beliefs you have collected over your lifetime. Many of those beliefs are not who you really are, but are based on *your* interpretation of how *others* see you. So, your subconscious is developed both from WHAT OTHERS SAY TO YOU, *and* WHAT YOU SAY TO YOURSELF. If those beliefs are experienced often enough, you will become the person you believe others think you are. Negative childhood programming from others, and your own negative thinking can mold your adult thinking. *Three examples are:*

- A child may be scolded continually by the mother for being slow. The mother may be tense and constantly overextended. The child may not be *unusually* slow at all. However, the child will grow up thinking he or she is slow because the mother firmly implanted the thought. Symptoms like low productivity, indecision, habitual tardiness, and slow reaction time, may appear as the child grows.

- A child may feel intellectually inferior being compared to a bright sibling. In high school, I was frequently referred to as *Lawrence's sister.* Since I did not think I could compete with my brother's intelligence, I decided to play a lighthearted clown role to avoid comparison. Blocking my intellectual awareness followed me for years. I performed well, but my belief system prevented me from acknowledging my accomplishments. It took years of working on self-esteem to overcome this inhibiting behavior.

- A child who feels unloved might grow up too involved in the PROCESS of looking for love, to

9

recognize love if it occurs. He or she might also get involved in a problem relationship because of the belief they do not deserve better. A person who did not feel special as a child, or felt unloved, may wonder who would care. Daily negative choices will set him or her up to continue the negative belief that *I can't be happy and life is hard... **and each relationship will confirm that belief system.***

You also have a creative subconscious that is the REAL you! But creativity can only be developed with positive thoughts; you cannot be creative with negative energy. You cannot always control what others say to you, but YOU CAN ALWAYS CONTROL WHAT YOU SAY TO YOURSELF! The more POSITIVE you think, the less likely you will continue to be influenced by your interpretation of negative childhood experiences. You are now *free* to make choices that will develop the creative YOU TODAY!

Jess Lair in his book I AIN'T MUCH BABY, BUT I'M ALL I'VE GOT, feels the best psychology he has found in 45 years of research is:

"YOU CAN SOLVE ALL YOUR PROBLEMS THAT CAN BE SOLVED BY GOING IN SEARCH OF THE MAGNIFICENT 'YOU', AND AN ADDED REWARD FOR THAT IS THE ACCEPTANCE OF OTHERS WHICH FREES THEM TO SEARCH FOR THEMSELVES, TOO."

SYMBIOTIC RELATIONSHIPS

All personality is not hereditary; much is a learned behavior. As children, we constantly want to please, and we quickly learn what behaviors are expected from us. We often suppress our own personality, if it conflicts with what we think others want us to be. The result is an internal tug-of-war that can continue for life. Many adults with suppressed personalities had at least one very dominant parent.

In a single parent home, a child may try even harder to please the remaining parent. A child may not develop decision-making normally if the parent has a controlling personality, and takes charge too often. When the child becomes an adult, he or she may have problems with productivity, creativity, and self-image. This usually surfaces as a real problem about mid-life when that adult realizes the need to feel in charge of his or her life. It is one reason some people make drastic changes in careers, relationships, and personal appearance during this period of their lives.

We often marry, or develop partnerships to strengthen our own weaknesses. Instead of two people being individuals, they combine to make up one personality. This process is called SYMBIOSIS, and is another cause of mid-life crisis. *For mental and emotional health, a person needs full development of the personality's three aspects:*

- the child state (ability to have fun)
- the parent state (ability to take care of oneself)
- the adult state (intellectual development)

One reason we have negative thoughts about ourselves is because we see our own weaknesses. We all want to feel confident, responsible, intelligent, and willing to have fun. We all want to be in charge of our child, parent and adult states. We may not know what is missing in those words, but we experience an unhappy feeling about ourselves. Searching for mental and emotional peace can become very frustrating without the right knowledge to guide you.

In the positive use of symbiosis, neither consenting person is harmed; the association can be beneficial to both. What happens too often, is the basic human need to feel like a WHOLE, CAPABLE PERSON is not being satisfied for one of the participants. This now unsatisfied basic need irritates that person into resenting the association. Now the union is not beneficial, and marital or partnership problems develop. For example, a young man with a poor child state marries a fun-loving girl, who in mid-life decides to develop a more serious intellectual side. The man may not appreciate the wife's new image, if he is still lacking a child state. She has developed her personality; he resents her growth because he is still the same.

Many people simply do not know how to have fun; they have an undeveloped child state. Growing up with a struggling single parent, financial hardship, or family disaster can damage one's child state. Life was hard for the child. As an adult, his or her belief confirms that life is hard, by being unwilling to have fun. They become couch potatoes, victims, introverts, or "bah humbug" year round.

WAYS TO UNBLOCK YOUR CREATIVITY

Creativity can be one of the most enjoyable ways to put fun in a person's life. It can make a career stimulating, raising children more fun, and provide productive ways of filling time. It is a sad waste when a person's natural ability to be creative is blocked by negative subconscious beliefs. If your subconscious holds doubts about your intelligence, talent, or leadership qualities, you may go through life holding back, and have one disappointment after another.

You can decide *today* how you want to see yourself, and how you wish others to see you. To change your image, you need to reprogram your subconscious, and let that wonderful unblocked creativity take over. *You can do this by using the following techniques:*

*   **Deep relaxation tapes** are available through some health food stores, some bookstores, and health magazines.

*   **Counseling** needs careful consideration! Find a counselor who deals with the issues in a positive, forward energy, and does not keep you locked in the past.

12

*   **Neurolinguistic Programming (NLP)** is a technique that assists you in communicating with your subconscious, and changing whatever is needed to gain control over your life. It also assists you in communicating with others. Check a bookstore for books available to teach yourself the techniques.

*   **Affirmations** are positive thoughts you choose to put in your conscious mind. If you *repeat the affirmation often enough,* the positive information will be stored in your subconscious, and you will begin to believe it is true.

    You become what you *think* you are. If you think you are successful, then you become successful. If you think you are stupid, or slow, then you become stupid or slow. The words you use to describe yourself are very powerful ... SO STOP THE STINKING THINKING! You either program yourself, or are influenced by other people's thoughts or words. Your mind controls your actions, emotions, and attitudes, based on the information it receives. *So, if you keep telling your mind you cannot do anything right, is it surprising that you will find yourself doing everything wrong?* Use positive words to change bad habits, establish new ones, and develop new patterns of behavior.

    Affirmations greatly assist a person with an intense determination to change. *Try these techniques:*

    -   **Personalize the affirmation** by saying, "I, (name), am successful."

    -   **Acknowledge other people have conditioned you.** Look into a mirror and say, "You, (name), are successful." Eye to eye contact in the mirror directs the affirmation to you. Whenever possible, use your mirror.

    -   **State your affirmations in the present tense,** as though you have already achieved your goal. For example, never say, "I plan to become successful." This gives you an excuse for not being successful NOW. Instead say, "I AM successful!" Remember, you are *developing* a **POSITIVE BELIEF SYSTEM** that will help you make choices to support your new beliefs.

- **State your affirmations in the positive form.** Instead of saying, "I do not want to smoke," say, "I, (name), make healthy choices for my well being."

- **Repeat your affirmation throughout the day.** Your brain will eventually get the message, and will believe anything you tell it often enough. State your affirmations when you first get up, as often as possible throughout the day, and the last thing before retiring. Put signs in the bathroom, on the refrigerator, and in your car to remind you to say them often.

   I was stating my "successful" affirmation waiting for a red light to change. It reminded me to call a contact I knew about for months. I called when I got home. The effort resulted in a professional opportunity, plus a radio and a television interview. ***POSITIVE AFFIRMATIONS HELP KEEP YOU ACTION ORIENTED!***

- **Be firm and do not stop just because you do not believe it yet.** You may laugh when you look in the mirror and say, "I, (name), am beautiful." That will not prevent exciting changes from occurring if you keep saying it. You will become motivated to make those changes, and you will learn to see yourself in a different way. You will start to like yourself more, and see beauty as more than surface appearance. You may decide to make changes that could improve the way you physically look to yourself and others.

Affirmations can be acting rather than verbal. If you wake up some morning feeling depressed or irritable, force yourself to be pleasant to the first person you see. You will find your whole attitude changing. You can *choose* to stay depressed or irritable, BUT WHAT A WASTE OF ENERGY THAT IS!!!

Changing the subconscious mind needs as much positive repetition as you gave negative thoughts before. Most health food stores carry **BACH FLOWER REMEDIES** that assist in changing from negative to positive thoughts and feelings through repetitious positive affirmations. Check the Resource References for books on Bach Flowers. The different Bach Flower Remedies are worth listing here. The negative feelings are listed first, followed by a suggested positive affirmation; or you may choose your own words. *You must state a positive affirmation each time you take the remedy.* Do you recognize yourself in any of the following?

AGRIMONY -- Attempts to conceal disturbing thoughts behind a façade of cheerfulness.
  "I am finding peace within myself."

ASPEN - Apprehensions, fear of some impending evil.
  "I feel confident and strong."

BEECH – Arrogance, intolerance, criticizing without understanding of the views of others.
  "I am making peace with myself and others."

CENTUARY – Weak-willed, easily exploited, can't say no.
  "I stand up for my own needs."

CERATO – Doubting own judgement, and having to seek the confirmation of others.
"Only I can decide what is right for me."

CHERRY PLUM – Fear of letting go, fear of losing control, uncontrollable bursts of anger.
"I accept my calm inner guidance."

CHESTNUT BUD – Repeating the same faults over and over due to lack of learning from experiences.
"I am learning something from every experience."

CHICORY – Possessive, interfering, manipulating the affairs of others, self-pity, demanding full support from others.
"I respect the boundaries of every individual."

CLEMATIS – Daydreaming, paying little attention to what is going on around you.
"I am attentive to what is happening now."

CRAB APPLE - Feeling of being unclean, infected, inner disgust with self.
"I am at peace with my mind and body."

ELM – Overwhelmed by responsibility.
"I do the best I can at any given time."

GENTIAN – Skeptical, pessimistic, easily discouraged.
"Obstacles are opportunities to learn."

GORSE – Long term suffering from chronic disease that produces negative expectations, and reinforces disease.
"Hope brings healing energy."

HEATHER – Needs an audience to express in detail everything that happens.
"I am secure within myself."

HOLLY – Hatred, envy, jealousy, suspicion.
"I concentrate on my own personal development."

HONEYSUCKLE – Clings to the past.
"I release the past, and make myself available in the present."

HORNBEAM – Weariness and exhaustion is largely in the mind.
"I feel awake and refreshed."

IMPATIENS – Impatient, intolerant, irritable.
"Each part of my journey as its own speed."

LARCH-Lack of self-confidence, and fear of failure.
"I can do it; I will do it; I am doing it."

MIMULUS – Shy, timid, fearful.
"My inner strength and courage releases my fear."

MUSTARD – Dark cloud feeling that saddens for no known reason, or powerless feeling.
"My heart feels light and hopeful."

OAK – Never knowing when to let go of the fight against great odds.
"I know it is time to move on in my life."

OLIVE – Exhaustion, drained energy on the physical level.
"I feel energy flowing into me."

PINE – Guilt complex blaming self even for the mistakes of others.
"I forgive and love myself."

RED CHESTNUT – Excessive concern over others.
"I radiate optimism, and allow others to live their journey."

ROCK WATER – Life's pleasures are suffocated under self-imposed disciplines.
"I am open to new insights and experiences."

ROCK ROSE - Acute state of fear, terror, panic.
"I am in God's hands."

SCLERANTHUS – Indecisive, erratic, fluctuating moods.
"The definite decision is within me."

STAR OF BETHLEHEM – Paralyzing sorrow following shocking events.
"My whole system is calmly breathing."

SWEET CHESTNUT – Hopeless despair; reached the limit of endurance.
"Night has to come before it can be day again."

VERVAIN – Overly enthusiastic, even fanatical.
"I control my energy, and learn from others."

VINE – Dominating, inflexible, striving for power.
"I learn from the uniqueness of every individual."

WALNUT – Difficulties in adjusting to life's changes; need protecting from outside influences.

18

"I dismiss limiting factors that inhibit my journey."

WATER VIOLET – Loners who need to be alone with little emotional involvement.
"I need the world, and the world needs me."

WHITE CHESTNUT – Unwanted thoughts keep going around in one's head.
"The solutions I need will come to mind."

WILD OAT – Dissatisfaction with one's mission in life.
"I allow my life journey to guide me in my growth."

WILD ROSE – Resignation, lack of ambition, apathy.
"Life is getting more interesting and beautiful."

WILLOW – Unspoken resentment, bitterness, and victim attitude.
"I am thinking, doing, and achieving positive things."

Bach Flower Remedies do not change the situation. They change your interpretation of the situation. Now, those positive interpretations can help you do things differently ... *and that can change the situation.*

[] [] [] [] [] []

Have you ever listened carefully to someone with a negative attitude? Try it sometime, and recall the words or phrases they use most often. *You will hear a lot of words like:*

I want to, but	perhaps	so-so
I hope so	maybe	I don't know
I wish I could	later	I can't help it
I plan to someday	I'll try	possibly

These negative people exhaust their energy. "I am trying," means nothing. You either ARE, or you ARE NOT making your life work for you. Change your vocabulary, and imagine what your day could be like. The reward for hanging on to negative words is AVOIDANCE; you do not have to deal with challenge. You start the day with all your "comfort zones," and end the day with *lost opportunities* to learn and enjoy life.

Replace negative words with positive words like:

I will	yes	I would love to
I do	now	that's exciting
I can	definitely	I care
let's go	I'll help	certainly

You may believe negative things about yourself, and you will act accordingly to confirm these negative beliefs ... TIME AND TIME AGAIN! If you can admit your own negative thoughts, you can now CONSCIOUSLY choose to change your thoughts and attitude.

Shyness is a widespread psychological problem of Americans today. Picture yourself as you would like to be ... then practice positive affirmations. You must first communicate with *yourself*, before you will successfully venture out and be comfortable with *others*.

THE THREE WAYS TO REPROGRAM THE SUBCONSCIOUS ARE:

-   **POSITIVE AFFIRMATIONS** - I AM SOMETHING, AND I WILL MAKE THE MOST OF THAT SOMETHING, is a good positive affirmation.

-   **WILL AND DETERMINATION** - You simply have had enough of the way your life has been going, and you WILL make it better!!!

-   **USE THE WORD "OR" TO CHANGE NEGATIVE WORDS OR THOUGHTS TO POSITIVE WORDS OR THOUGHTS** - As soon as you say or think, "I will never learn that," follow it immediately with, "Or, I will." Listen to your own words or thoughts. *You may be surprised how often you sabotage your day ... all by yourself!*

[] [] [] [] [] []

PAYOFFS FOR HANGING ON TO ILLNESS

No one wants to be sick or unmotivated; there has to be some kind of a *pay-off* for a person to hang on to illness. People want to be healthy and successful ... unless, of course, they do not. If this is the case, something in the negative subconscious is getting satisfied. I will qualify this by saying continuous stress may have created minor symptoms at first. However, treating only the symptoms without getting to the cause of the problems can lead to more stress, and more symptoms. Then, poor diet choices, nutritional deficiencies, allergies, chemical sensitivities, hiding out in addictive habits, taking unnecessary drugs with multiple side effects, or not living by "laws" that promote health can make simple symptoms into out-of-control symptoms. The person may now be sick on all levels of spiritual, mental,

21

emotional, and physical. HOW IT ALL GOT STARTED IS LOST IN WHAT HAS NOW BECOME A CRISIS.

A person with negative subconscious beliefs will usually make a lot of wrong health choices. Their deteriorating health keeps them in the VICTIM state. They actually become *comfortable in their discomfort.* For them, the *pay-off* is **CONFIRMING** that *I can't be happy ... or life is hard.* ***People survive in their conscious thoughts. They may be unaware that their negative subconscious drives them.***

> *One example is a woman who got married young, and did not develop her own identity while staying home to take care of a family. On a "conscious" level she thought she was happy living the affluent American dream. Her daily choices produced negative health results. Something was wrong with her dream life! Her loss of **potential** and **personal** development set her up for ill health. The subconscious belief of feeling incomplete can be suppressed, because we too often value the materialistic present instead of self-growth.*

WHY DO PEOPLE WHO TRULY BELIEVE THEY WOULD LIKE TO BE HEALTHY CONTINUE TO EXPERIENCE POOR HEALTH? Have you ever sat down to evaluate yourself, and *decided you needed to lie down*? If so, understanding how payoffs influence your life could help you evaluate the choices you make ... and that is a place to start!

Here are just a few examples of payoffs:

- **TO AVOID INTIMACY** - Using the old saying, "Not now, I've got a headache," has been expanded to include backache, stomachache, muscle pain and other body symptoms. It works every time, because our society is very "symptom" oriented. Poor health is used successfully to keep people away.

- **GETTING THE JOB YOU WANT** - Poor health can get you changed from a job you do not like, to one you prefer. You may keep a backache until you get the sit-down job you wanted. You may stay unemployed or plagued with problems, because that confirms your belief that you are not capable of success.

- **TO AVOID RESPONSIBILITY** - If you are afraid of competing or assuming responsibility, you may become introverted. People are not born shy. They get that way because there is a pay-off confirming a belief that they are weak and unimportant.

[] [] [] [] [] []

MINDTRAPS KEEP YOU LOCKED IN THE PAST

Your state of mind has much to do with your control over life. The way you respond to any situation is your reaction based on the beliefs in your subconscious mind. This reaction, called a **MINDTRAP**, is the way you deal with suppressed fear and insecurity. *Mindtraps keep you locked in suppressed trauma or negative childhood teachings.* Accept the past for the good and the bad in it ... then go on with your life. You cannot undo the past, but you can accept it, and learn from past experiences to make you stronger. **YOU** are now in charge of the present and the future. Acknowledging a mindtrap is a start to understanding what you are suppressing. *Mindtraps prevent you from coping with:*

- **THE PRESENT** - Living in the past is easier than challenging the present, and you never have to develop your potential.

- **SUPPRESSED TRAUMA** - You stay locked in, and haunted by past negative experiences.

23

- **NEGATIVE CHILDHOOD TEACHINGS** - You go internal, and do not give yourself credit for being in control *now*.

In his book, MAKING CONTACT: A GUIDE TO OVERCOMING SHYNESS, Arthur Wassner states:

"SHYNESS MAY BE THE MOST WIDESPREAD AND LEAST NOTICED PSYCHOLOGICAL PROBLEM OF AMERICANS TODAY."

WHAT ARE SOME EXAMPLES OF MINDTRAPS?

- **GUILT** – You are feeling guilty about everything. "I'm sure I'm the one to blame." "I'm the one who causes all the trouble." You apologize constantly. Suppressed trauma like this can occur from guilt over injuring a loved one, parent's divorce, or other family crisis you caused ... or think you caused.

- **MISTRUST** - You do not trust love, friendship, job security, or anything else. Childhood abuse, physical or emotional neglect, or abandonment can result in serious mistrust.

- **CONFUSION** - In childhood you may have felt incompetent, so living in chaos keeps people from giving you responsibility.

- **DEFENSIVENESS** - Physical or verbal harassment in childhood produces this mindtrap.

- **SHAME** - This mindtrap can result from poor handling by adults of childhood events, like stealing or sexual issues.

- **RATIONALIZATION** - This excuses one's conscious act without realizing the real subconscious motive. "It is okay to lie if it helps you get ahead." You feel driven to act in a certain way. You may not *consciously* acknowledge the driving force from the past.

There are many mindtraps like regret, humiliation, emptiness, resentment, resignation, explanation, self-righteousness, and others. Remember, for better or for worse, the past was part of your life. Accept it was your *past*. Now you can be in charge of the *present* and the *future*. *You do not have to live in a world of mindtraps.*

[] [] [] [] [] []

BOTH BEHAVIOR AND FEELINGS COME FROM YOUR BELIEFS. IF YOU DO NOT LIKE THE WAY YOUR LIFE IS GOING, ASK YOURSELF:

- **IS THERE A GOOD REASON FOR MY BELIEF?** If so, are you letting a past experience you had no control over affect today, which you DO have control over? *Consider this story:*

    A baby circus elephant is restrained with a well-secured chain. He struggles but cannot get free. As he grows, the secured chain is changed to bigger and stronger. After a while, believing he cannot get loose, he stops struggling. A huge elephant in the circus is restrained with only a small peg in the ground. Many adults behave like the circus elephant, restrained in thought and action all their lives based on a belief system.

- **COULD I BE MISTAKEN IN MY BELIEF?** Could your interpretation of the situation be changed with more understanding, compassion, or change in attitude?

- **EVEN IF MY BELIEF IS TRUE, SHOULD I CONTINUE LETTING IT INFLUENCE MY LIFE?**

25

"I'M NOT FREE UNTIL I BELIEVE IN ME."

- Robert H. Schuller

- **DO I REALLY HAVE A COMMITMENT TO IMPROVE THE QUALITY OF MY LIFE?** *IF NOT ... WHY WOULD I WANT TO LIVE EACH DAY THE SAME AS BEFORE?*

[] [] [] [] [] []

WAYS TO ENHANCE YOUR POTENTIAL

Everyone has the power within himself or herself to produce a giant. Most people only use a fraction of their capabilities. To create a better self-image does not create NEW abilities ... it RELEASES the ones you already have! *To enhance your potential:*

1. **PARTICIPATE in life 100 percent rather than living as an observer ...** GET ACTIVE! Procrastination is the art of keeping up with yesterday. It is all right to be lazy occasionally. This may sound like a paradox, but a person works best who can relax enough to assimilate daily experiences, renew their energy and take time to plan. *The word is BALANCE.*

   "THERE ARE NO RULES HERE; WE'RE TRYING TO GET SOMETHING DONE."

   - Thomas Edison

2. **BE HONEST with yourself and others,** if you expect others to be honest with you. *If you tell the truth, you do not have to remember anything.*

26

3. **TRUST your own judgment.** Make a list of your best qualities, and do not be afraid to pat yourself on the back!

4. **ACCEPT other points of view.** Unless you listen to what someone else says, you can only base your opinion on what you THINK you know. Do not be so hard on yourself in a learning situation. Everyone is ignorant ... only on different subjects.

5. **COMMUNICATE with people.** Observe people's response to how you speak to them. Be clear and concise so people do not just hear what you say, but understand what you mean. The following two statements, "You have a face that could stop a clock," and "When I look at you time stands still," have the same meaning, but can be interpreted very differently.

6. **SUPPORT others to win in life.** Everyone loves a supporter. Share your experiences; be a good listener. Act as if other people are important.

> *"I CAN GO TWO WEEKS WITH ONE COMPLIMENT FROM A FRIEND."*
>
> - Mark Twain

To handle yourself, use your head; to handle others, use your heart.

> *"BE SOMEONE FOR SOMEBODY."*
>
> - Mother Teresa

7. **DO NOT LIVE IN DAILY JUDGMENT of others.** You do not know all the facts about another person's life, so you cannot **accurately** assess how their experiences have affected them. Everyone does the best

they can at any given time. Just like you, they may have had many experiences that left scars. Not everyone has the opportunity to learn what makes them think, feel, or act the way they do ... so ... THEY DO THE BEST THEY CAN DO AT THE TIME! Do not try to change anyone but yourself! You will like, or understand almost everyone you meet better, after you get to know them.

> *"I AM POSITIVELY ADDICTED TO GIVING PEOPLE HOPE."*

> - Robert H. Schuller

8. **FORGIVE who you are angry at;** they did the best they could do at the time. Then forgive yourself for reacting. Understand that nobody is perfect, including you. Allow other people to have *their* journey!

A shocking part of society has turned downright vicious, but many people are still gentle. This beautifully written book preface about gentle people trying to survive in a dog-eat-dog world, is a favorite of mine, and well worth sharing.

> *This is a book born in my heart, born in the pain of ending one life and beginning another, born in the excitement of the continuing search for life's meaning. Some people do not have to search, they find their niche early in life and rest there, seemingly contented and resigned. They do not seem to ask much of life, sometimes they do not seem to take it seriously. At times I envy them, but usually I do not understand them. Seldom do they understand me.*

> *I am one of the searchers. There are, I believe, millions of us. We are not unhappy, but neither are we really content. We continue to explore life, hoping to uncover its ultimate secret. We continue to explore ourselves, hoping to understand. We like to walk along*

28

the beach, we are drawn by the ocean, taken by its power, its unceasing motion, its mystery and unspeakable beauty. We like forests and mountains, deserts and hidden rivers, and the lonely cities as well. Our sadness is as much a part of our lives as is our laughter. To share our sadness with one we love is perhaps as great a joy as we can know – unless it be to share our laughter.

We searchers are ambitious only for life itself, for everything beautiful it can provide. Most of all we want to love and be loved. We want to live in a relationship that will not impede our wondering, nor prevent our search, nor lock us in prison walls, that will take us for what little we have to give. We do not want to prove ourselves to another or to compete for love.

This is a book for wanderers, dreamers and lovers, for lonely men and women who dare to ask of life everything good and beautiful. It is for those who are too gentle to live among wolves.

- James Kavanaugh

9. **Understand that TOUCH is an exchange of "energy."** Energy is what makes the world go round. "Reach out and touch someone" is more than a telephone commercial. A touch is worth a thousand words because it means what life is all about ... caring. Touchers are usually less afraid, less tense, and less suspicious of others. Non-touchers tend to be more internal, unstable, apprehensive, and usually have low self-esteem.

10. **BE YOURSELF;** dump phony images. Admit you are flawed, but you are becoming ... !

"KNOW YOURSELF! DON'T ACCEPT YOUR DOG'S ADMIRATION AS CONCLUSIVE EVIDENCE THAT YOU ARE WONDERFUL."

- Ann Landers

11. **BE FLEXIBLE** and willing to try something else, if what you want out of life is not happening. Just because it is a well-worn path, does not mean it is the right one. Commit yourself to your belief system ... if it works for you. Be willing to change if it does not work for you.

"THIS TIME, LIKE ALL OTHER TIMES, IS A VERY GOOD ONE, IF WE BUT KNEW WHAT TO DO WITH IT."
- Ralph Waldo Emerson

12. **LOVE YOURSELF.** If you do not love yourself, why should anyone else love you? It is necessary to recognize your shortcomings, but disastrous to hate yourself for them. YOU ARE GREAT ... AND GETTING BETTER! Give yourself credit for each small success. With self-confidence comes leadership ... and with leadership comes charisma. **Charisma is just an attitude of confidence!**

"WHO YOU REALLY ARE IS NOT A COLLECTION OF PARTS BUT A WHOLE. SEEING YOURSELF AS WHOLE IS THE FIRST STEP TOWARDS SEEING YOURSELF AS TRULY ATTRACTIVE."
- Deepak Chopra

13. **HAVE FUN!** Learn to live life in the experiential sensory groups: visual (sight), auditory (hearing), kinesthetic (feeling), gustatory (taste), and olfactory

30

(smell). Tuning out any one listed diminishes your awareness. In our society …

- sight is often tuned out. Your home may not be what you want, or you do not enjoy your personal appearance.

- a noisy neighborhood, job, or noisy children, may make you tune out hearing.

- avoidance of intimacy or traumatic emotional crisis can make you tune out feeling.

- people living with animals, or strong continuous odor from air or living conditions, often block out smell.

Blocking sensory experiences diminishes your awareness, and that can reduce opportunities that could add pleasure to your life. Think of going to the mountains, **SEEING** the spectacular view, **HEARING** the wind and water, **SMELLING** the woods aroma, **FEELING** a soft velvet flower, and **TASTING** your delicious lunch. That sort of *complete* sensory experience is what having fun, and enjoying life is all about.

We should not have to look back on the "carefree days of childhood" as though they are completely gone. Some adults never allow themselves that sort of non-goal directed behavior. Some adults are always trying to accomplish something. It is not important what you play … IT IS JUST IMPORTANT THAT YOU PLAY! Growing up for some people is not fun. What they do not realize is that *if they had not lost the ability to play along the way,* life might have been easier. Perhaps the single most outstanding characteristic of healthy people is their SENSE OF HUMOR.

14. **LEARN about your behavior** by observing how you respond to situations. If you smoke or eat every time you get tense, the negative addiction will be very hard to break because it not only pacifies the struggle, but also actually provides pleasurable experience. You substitute pleasure for the stress, and accept that it is all right because you enjoy it so much. Smokers like to smoke ... overeaters like to eat ... drinkers like to drink. *This enjoyment prevents you from facing the REASON for the addiction ... what you are NOT getting.*

Keep promises and be reliable; be on time for appointments. If this is a problem, you need to look for a mindtrap, or a pay-off.

15. **BE ACCOUNTABLE for what you do.** The greatest fault is to be conscious of none.

16. **COMMIT to winning in life.** This does not necessarily imply financial or career success; winning in life means being the best in whatever is most important to you.

IF YOU WANT TO DO IT ... DO IT!
IF YOU WANT TO LEARN IT ... LEARN IT!
ONLY YOU CAN STOP YOUR CREATIVITY
WHICH IS ALREADY THERE!

"THE MOST GLORIOUS MOMENTS IN YOUR LIFE ARE NOT THE SO-CALLED DAYS OF SUCCESS, BUT RATHER THOSE DAYS WHEN OUT OF DEJECTION AND DESPAIR, YOU FEEL RISE IN YOU A CHALLENGE TO LIFE, AND THE PROMISE OF FUTURE ACCOMPLISHMENTS."

- Gustave Flaubert

The three C's - commitment, control, and challenge are the ingredients of "hardiness." Hardy people face change with confidence; less hardy people feel threatened. Hardy people stay healthier, even if they have a strong family history of disease.

Sir Ernest Shackleton ran this ad in a London paper for an Antarctic expedition:

> *MEN WANTED FOR HAZARDOUS JOURNEY, SMALL WAGES, BITTER COLD, LONG MONTHS OF COMPLETE DARKNESS, CONSTANT DANGER, SAFE RETURN DOUBTFUL. HONOR AND RECOGNITION IN CASE OF SUCCESS."*

When all returned alive, he wrote:

> *"WE PIERCED THE VENEER OF OUTSIDE THINGS, AND REACHED THE NAKED SOUL OF MAN."*

How can you learn to be hardy? **By viewing daily stressors in ways that produce MINIMAL stress response.** A person of conviction must either choose one side of the road or the other ... not the middle of the road ... or on the fence! Few people today reach the depth of human satisfaction that is the ultimate of hardiness. In our soft, modern ways we have forgotten how to be tough enough to reach our naked soul.

Too often we:

- play it safe
- aim for the sure thing
- want life to be easy
- seldom stretch ourselves

17. **CELEBRATE LIFE each day.** *Even with daily problems and challenges, you should enjoy the experience of living.* If you do not agree with that, you need to read the rest of this book, and live by the "laws" of wellness long enough for your physical body to heal.

Healing your mental and emotional state is largely based on "attitude."

Your Creator has a plan for you. Concentrate on the two reasons you are here on earth:

- to learn and grow
- to be in service to humankind

"I WAS RICH, IF NOT IN MONEY, IN SUNNY HOURS AND SUMMER DAYS."

- Henry David Thoreau

I wrote a poem about enjoying life:

JOYFUL DAY

The day begins
The dawn arrives
Down around my face
supplies my needs.
Sunbeams invite me
Song birds delight me
Oh day, JOYFUL DAY.

Another day the clouds appear
The rain drowns out the birds I hear.
No matter,
I still have the sun in me.
Oh day, JOYFUL DAY!

18. **BE RECEPTIVE to new ideas.** New ideas can create a sense of being fearful. Fear is a limiting belief that keeps you from what you want. If you learn more about what you fear, you will reduce or eliminate the fear. Do not be afraid of a challenge. What you do not know, you can always learn.

Snake handlers do not fear poisonous snakes because they learned how to respect and handle them. They traded fear for knowledge.

Your life journey should be an exciting journey. Change is good, but to enjoy life to the fullest, remember balance. We need both paved highways, and trails through quiet woods. We can enjoy television, but also enjoy time to see flying geese in the fall.

[] [] [] [] [] []

In the movie about Eleanor Roosevelt, she said, "FEAR IS AN ILLUSION. IF YOU PUT THE SAME ENERGY IN CONFIDENCE, THE MOST WONDERFUL THINGS HAPPEN." Eleanor Roosevelt's life was filled with accomplishments, because she had a positive attitude. If you approach every day, every task, and every goal with the same enthusiasm, you too can accomplish "wonderful things" ...
CHALLENGE YOURSELF!

A personal fear was challenged by signing up for a two-day raft trip without the support of my husband. Beneath my fascination with rafting was a genuine fear of the water. The orientation included a whitewater movie that left me sinking into my chair. By the end of the film I left fingernail marks on the man next to me. He was so scared he did not feel anything.

We were instructed to dress in light layers. I was so sure I would end up in the cold water, I wore long underwear and warm ski clothes. I looked pretty strange crawling into the boat next to people in bathing suits. The black electric tape someone gave me to secure my glasses was disturbing to me, since a class on colors suggested black was not my best color.

The adventure ran me through the whole gamut of emotions from abject terror to pride. Emotions by the end of the day were both excitement and relief; I had actually survived. By the end of the second day (in my bathing suit), fulfillment was overwhelming. Respect for the river had replaced fear. Satisfaction had replaced wishful thinking. I had challenged more than the river. I had challenged myself.

By confronting one fear, it would be easier to confront others. I used to think I had to have someone with me for support. I had someone this time ... myself! In the future, my positive energy will be reinforced by new confidence. Discovering the joys of living with a beginner's mind is no longer a problem.

I am not suggesting that you challenge every fear you have. I do not choose to skydive or climb rocks, so those fears do not contain negative energy. Any situation you would like to participate in, but are afraid to, contains negative energy. If you put that energy into confidence, and *learn what you need to learn* ... **you open the door for the most wonderful things to happen!**

[] [] [] [] [] []

Experience, good or bad, is both an event you learn from, and what you *do* with what happened to you. The source of experience is what is happening WITHIN you, not the actual event. No event or series of events should control what a person becomes. That should be under his or her control ... thus, experience results from one's *handling* of life's joys, triumphs, sorrows, and defeats.

The question is not, "ARE YOU PERFECT?" ... but, "ARE YOU LEARNING FROM YOUR MISTAKES?"

In his senior year in high school, my youngest son's baseball team was hoping to be in the championship series, when they lost an early game in the third extra inning. Frustrated, my son slammed his fist towards the side of the dugout, but hit the drainpipe instead and broke his hand. He could have gone into depression, or played on the sympathy

36

of this teammates and family, but he chose differently. He accepted the situation with maturity and accountability. He spent the rest of the season in a cast, but was such a team booster he got the Most Inspirational Player award, and a $500 college scholarship for Best All-Around Team Member. That boost to his self-esteem set the groundwork for his whole life.

The experience, for him, was not the broken hand; it was the opportunity to accept a difficult situation (*which was the outcome of his own actions*), and make it a positive experience. He learned some valuable character traits can be built out of adversity.

[] [] [] [] [] []

If you do not like the way you are, YOU HAVE THE POWER TO CHANGE YOURSELF. You should not believe you have the right to change others. Learn to enjoy the people around you for who they are. You have to deal with many different people in life. You will only frustrate yourself if you can not accept each one for their own uniqueness. *Possibility thinking is different for everyone.*

What makes people act the way they do? Why do they act differently than you? We all belong, in one way or another, to different personality groups. *The four basic groups are: ANALYST, SUPPORTER, CONTROLLER, and PROMOTER.* You may have traits in all four groups, or be strong in three, have a combination of two, or be intense in one. There is a positive and a negative side to each personality, and you will experience each at one time or another. Do not apologize because you clearly belong to any one group ... the truth is:

You are not *inferior*.
You are not *superior*.
You are simply *you*.

TO FIND YOUR DOMINANT PERSONALITY GROUP ASK IF:

MOST OF THE TIME *do you prefer to be in charge, or do you prefer someone else to be in charge?*

MOST OF THE TIME *are you formal in the precision of your work, or do you have a more relaxed attitude about details?*

Combine your answers in these various ways:

If you are NOT DOMINANT and FORMAL most of the time, you are an analyst.

If you are NOT DOMINANT and INFORMAL most of the time, you are a supporter.

If you are DOMINANT and FORMAL most of the time, you are a controller.

If you are DOMINANT and INFORMAL most of the time, you are a promoter.

You will enjoy your family, your co-workers, your friends, and even yourself more if you stretch out of your own quadrant into the quadrant of other people. Appreciate people for who *THEY* are. Share your talents, but do not force your beliefs on others. THERE ARE LESSONS TO BE LEARNED BY OBSERVING, RATHER THAN DOMINATING! *The one thing you should know for sure, is that there is an awful lot you do not know ... stretch yourself! Be willing to be **all** you can be!*

BASIC PERSONALITY GROUPS

ANALYST - NOT DOMINANT AND FORMAL

POSITIVE TRAITS	NEGATIVE TRAITS
Industrious	Critical/Picky
Persistent/enjoys learning	Indecisive/Resistant
Serious/Sensible	Moralistic/controls emotions
Exacting/Detailed	Stuffy
Orderly/Logical	Can overdo details
Data gathering	Reluctant initiative

SUPPORTER - NOT DOMINANT AND INFORMAL

POSITIVE TRAITS	NEGATIVE TRAITS
Pliable/Supportive	Moves slowly/Procrastinates
Enjoys people and family	Communicates poorly
Respectful	Unsure without direction
Willing/Agreeable	Needs timetable
Quick to accept	Can be wishy-washy
Conforming	Reluctant to be tough
Dependable	Needs precise information

CONTROLLER - DOMINANT AND FORMAL

POSITIVE TRAITS	NEGATIVE TRAITS
Strong-willed/Independent	Pushy/Dominating
Practical	Brusque/Severe/Harsh
Individualized	Expects much of others
Businesslike	Demanding
Decisive/Observant	Perfectionist
Efficient/Selective	May be too selective
Maximum potential	Speed too important

PROMOTER - DOMINANT AND INFORMAL

POSITIVE TRAITS	NEGATIVE TRAITS
Ambitious	Manipulative
Enthusiastic/Lots of hustle	Undisciplined/Impulsive
Friendly/Likes people	Egotistical
Communicates	Can be sloppy
Likes adventure	Can overlook fine points
Stimulating/Dramatic	Overly talkative/Excitable
Likes a challenge	Impatient

Understanding the personalities of people with whom you associate can be helpful in communicating with them. *Some examples are:*

- **CHILDREN -** I had an analyst child and a supporter child. If I had known this at critical times, I could have prevented *many* problems. Do not compare children; they are beautifully different. Allow children to be themselves, and not a forced carbon copy of you.

- **CO-WORKERS -** If you are unable to get along with a particular co-worker, information about his or her personality group can help you better understand how to be flexible in the situation.

- **STAFF -** Office staffing needs to be balanced. Two strong controllers in one area can be destructive. A whole office of strong controllers would be disastrous! A whole office of promoters want time to play. Supporters without leadership will not be able to make positive changes. Analysts will be so busy with details, that productivity could be reduced.

- **YOURSELF -** The negative side of your personality shows how you can create problems for yourself. It may also show that you are too dominant in one group. **The**

most balanced personality has some traits in each group.

I know a lady who was considered to be a supporter by her friends. She often appeared unhappy, and struggled with health issues. During a seminar she discovered that as a child, she did not want to grow up to be like her very strong, controlling mother. When she realized that it was possible to be a nice controller, she expanded her talents and assumed the more comfortable role of leadership. Her stress tolerance, and her health improved.

- **RELATIONSHIPS** - There are two combinations that typically tend to have problems relating. One is analyst/controller. The analyst wants all the data before making a decision, and is very irritating to the decisive controller. The other disastrous combination would be two inflexible controllers. Battle lines are drawn, and the fur flies.

COMBINATIONS THAT WORK WELL TOGETHER:

Two Analysts - They can get along amicably, but an excess of logic and order might make this relationship subdued!

A Supporter and an Analyst, or two Supporters - They make an effective team, but the relationship may lack spark. Supporters give support to any other personality.

A Promoter works well with all four personality groups - They add fun and excitement to the supporter or analyst's life.

Two FLEXIBLE Controllers - They can get along, as long as they allow each other equal time to be in control.

Many people received valuable lessons from their parents that set the stage for maturity. They become stronger from early lessons, and are ready to deal with life's challenges as their life evolves. Other people need to *find their strength* as an adult, because their childhood was filled with stress. *Knowing who you are helps you make the most of **today**.* Today is the most important day in your life ... yesterday is over, and tomorrow has not come. You can allow your past to keep you weak ... or you can become stronger from the worse of experiences.

"WHAT YOU ARE IS YOUR FOLK'S FAULT. BUT, IF YOU STAY THAT WAY, IT IS YOUR FAULT."

- unknown author in freshman psychology class

You are in charge of your life now. You are either thinking in a positive or negative way ... THERE IS NO ALMOST POSITIVE. We can program ourselves for failure by harping self-criticism and victim stories ... OR ... we can program ourselves for success by *TAKING CHARGE OF OUR ENERGY AND DOING SOMETHING POSITIVE WITH IT THROUGH ACTION!*

BE IN CHARGE OF YOUR
PERSONAL DEVELOPMENT

1. **STATE YOUR GOALS IN POSITIVE TERMS.** Let those goals be possible and practical; stay away from fantasy. The idea of marrying a wealthy person and spending the rest of your life traveling around the world, while possibly attractive, is not a realistic goal. Your personal goals should stimulate your creativity. THE IMPORTANT THING IS THAT YOU ARE INSPIRED ABOUT SOMETHING. Even long term goals need to be worked on day by day. *That gives you a reason to get the day started with enthusiasm.*

42

Stress management consultants all agree that a key element in stress mastery is assessing personal values and goals. Know where you've been (and learn from your experiences) ... where you are ... and where you are going. You will not always figure it out, but the puzzle should be taking shape. If you put pieces here and there without any idea what the puzzle will look like, you might find yourself unhappy with the finished picture. The "mid-life crisis" often happens because a person suddenly finds their life half over, and they do not like the picture.

> *"IF YOU GET WHERE YOU'RE GOING, WHERE WILL YOU BE?"*
>
> - Robert Schuller

Only you can maintain and affect the outcome of each goal. Do not make a goal so big you will give up; achieve it in stages you feel are possible. It keeps you feeling successful rather than discouraged. Do not forget to pat *yourself* on the back with each success. This is a prayer that got past around so many times, there is no way to know where it came from, but it is worth repeating about giving yourself credit ... no matter how small.

Dear Lord,

So far today, I am doing all right. I have not gossiped, lost my temper, been greedy, grumpy, nasty, selfish, or self indulgent. I have not whined, complained, cursed, or eaten any chocolate. I have not charged on my credit card. However, I am going to get out of bed in a few minutes, and I will need a lot more help after that.

2. **KNOW WHAT IT WILL TAKE TO MAKE YOU HAPPY.** If you get stuck, you have a choice ... DO SOMETHING DIFFERENT! You can only get stuck if you

are attached to form, which is *your opinion* of what is true. Form keeps you inflexible. If you are not attached to inhibiting beliefs, you are available for new experiences, like my raft trip.

YOUR QUEST TO DEVELOP POSITIVE ENERGY WILL BE MORE SUCCESSFUL IF YOU UNDERSTAND YOUR BASIC NEEDS:

* **THE NEED FOR LOVE** - Life's greatest happiness is to be convinced we are loved by our Creator, ourselves, and our world.

   "THERE IS THE SAME DIFFERENCE IN A PERSON BEFORE AND AFTER HE IS IN LOVE AS THERE IS IN AN UNLIGHTED LAMP AND ONE THAT IS BURNING. THE LAMP IS THERE AND IT WAS A GOOD LAMP, BUT NOW IT IS SHEDDING LIGHT, AND THAT IS ITS REAL FUNCTION."
   - Vincent Van Gogh

* **THE NEED FOR SECURITY** - Too often love is a game with the hope of winning the "big" prize ... security. You are the only person you can count on. *Develop your own independence* because what is true in your life today, may not be true tomorrow. *Are you just an unlit lamp, or are you fulfilling your potential?*

* **THE NEED FOR SELF-ESTEEM** - To feel good about your personal growth and contribution to mankind is as natural a basic need as breathing. *Are you just an unlit lamp, or are you glowing from your internal lights?*

   "Self-esteem isn't everything. It is just that there is nothing without it."
   - *Gloria Swanson*

* THE NEED FOR NEW EXPERIENCES - It is this drive that sometimes "makes me wonder why I got myself in this mess." When you stop searching for new experiences in life, you are in the process of dying. New experiences give life a spark, and a challenge.

* THE NEED FOR RECOGNITION - Be dynamic; dress to win, and turn yourself on!

Look into a mirror and say, "I am worthy of feeling healthy in my body, and feeling good about myself!" Consider getting color draped, and adding the energy of the best colors for your complexion to your new enthusiasm for life. Introducing exciting color in your life means introducing *energy!*

Our selection of color is an expression of our acceptance or rejection of ourselves. If a person projects himself or herself as successful, and if their surroundings are bright, they will carry that energy into the day's activities. Color has a powerful influence on our health from the energy of red, yellow and orange, to the mellow blue, turquoise and purple, and the neutral greens. The more creatively we use color in our food, clothing, and environment, the more natural energy we generate to help us develop spiritually, mentally, emotionally, and physically. Color is the essence of the vital force all around us.

Another way both men and women can treat themselves to a *self-esteem lift* is to do an exercise *face-lift*. Your skin tone improves dramatically as oxygen and circulation are increased. Muscles are strengthened to create a toned, lifted appearance. Your self-confidence and self-esteem soar, making you feel more youthful and attractive. I highly recommend facial exercise books, tapes, and videos be a part of everyone's anti-aging routine. There are many variations being introduced in the television media and health community, so you should have no trouble locating one.

* **THE NEED FOR CREATIVE EXPRESSION** - The only thing that stops your creativity is your negative thinking!

3. **BE WILLING TO TAKE SENSIBLE RISKS.** Imagine two poles; the left one is where you are, the right one is where you want to be. The space between may be full of worry, fear, and tension (like a big mud puddle that will make you dirty if you cross). All personal development requires a degree of courage.

> *"NOT RISKING IS THE SUREST WAY OF LOSING. YOU NEVER LEARN WHO YOU ARE, NEVER TEST YOUR POTENTIAL, NEVER STRETCH OR REACH. YOU BECOME COMFORTABLE WITH FEWER AND FEWER EXPERIENCES. YOUR WORLD SHRINKS AND YOU BECOME RIGID. YOU BECOME A VICTIM."*
>
> - Dr. David Viscott

There are no failures, only different outcomes. We may feel stupid and ashamed at times because society is obsessed with success. Failure is a *personal judgment* about an event. The way we cope with failure is what shapes us, *NOT* the failure itself. You cannot fail if you accomplish something. It may not be the outcome you originally wanted, but you did not fail if you learned not to do it that way again. Life is one continuous learning process. You look at negative experiences in a new light when you acknowledge they are opportunities for personal growth ... and you learn ... and you learn your whole life.

4. **KEEP ON OPERATING.** The only way you can fail is to quit! Learn from success AND disappointment; and know that disappointment is not the ONLY response you can have. No one can make you angry, sad, depressed, or discouraged but you. Your reaction is *your* choice! Do not blame

anyone else for *your* choice. You are the one who decides the course of your future, **from the negative or positive interpretation of your daily experiences.**

> *"SUCCESS IS NEVER FINAL, FAILURE IS NEVER FATAL, AND IN DISCOURAGEMENT IS THE WORD 'COURAGE'. IT IS COURAGE THAT COUNTS."*

> \- Winston Churchill

Some people might not go to work with a slight headache, but would go on a cruise with the flu. If your intentions are high enough, almost no circumstance will intervene. If your intentions are low enough, any circumstance will intervene. Sometimes we need a nudge to get going again. The following story gives me the perfect word when I need a nudge.

> *A farmer saw a lost horse. When he got on its back to take it home, he said "giddy-up." The horse chose its own direction, and after a while wandered into the grass. The farmer let the horse eat, then urged the horse to continue down the trail. This happened several times, and each time "giddy-up" was all the horse needed to get back on the path. Eventually, they ended up in the horse's own barn.*

It is alright to wander off the trail occasionally to rest, but to get anywhere, you will need to get back on the trail. Sometimes "giddy-up" is needed to get started again. *Staying off the trail to personal development may be comfortable, but it will never be exciting or rewarding.*

Until you decide to do something, you will accomplish nothing. When the alarm goes off in the morning you can think about getting up, say you will do it and almost get up, but until you put your feet on the floor, you are not underway! Optimism is fine, but you have to add ACTION.

A honeybee may love being a honeybee, *but will not make any honey without taking 3.4 million trips to flowers.*

5. **STRETCH SOME ASPECT OF YOUR BEHAVIOR EVERYDAY.** Use someone who is accomplished in your field of interest as a model. It is alright to copy successful techniques.

> *"I WILL PREPARE MYSELF AND PERHAPS MY TIME WILL COME."*
> - Abraham Lincoln

6. **USE AFFIRMATIONS TO CHANGE YOUR INTERNAL DIALOGUE TO POSITIVE.** What is true or real is not important. What is important is whether your reality, or life as you know it, is rewarding to you. The feelings you have, come from what you say to yourself.

7. **LEARN COMMUNICATIONS SKILLS.** Everyone communicates, influences, and manipulates at one time or another. More important awareness is how are you going to do it, and for what reason? If you are not getting your point across, you need to understand more about your belief system. You need to acknowledge the beliefs of the person to whom you are speaking. Communication means both speaking AND listening.

   Knowledge of communication skills can keep you from getting stuck in a conversation that can lead to anger. Anger does not deserve to be judged harshly. It is just an emotion, like love, joy, and grief. Emotions are neither good nor bad. It is what you do with them that makes them good or bad!!

   A supporting slogan is, "I HAVE AN ABSOLUTE RIGHT TO BE WHO I AM, TO THINK WHAT I THINK, FEEL WHAT I FEEL, AND WANT WHAT I WANT." However, do not confuse "assertiveness" (your right to communicate your feelings) with "aggressiveness" (blaming others and judging their beliefs).

THE TWO MOST COMMON WAYS OF EXPRESSING ANGER IN AN UNHEALTHY WAY ARE:

- Misdirected anger can cause you to "kick the cat" because you are angry at your spouse. Burying the real problem just creates more problems.

- Complete suppression is very damaging because once you suppress one emotion, you begin to suppress them all.

WHAT HAPPENS WHEN ANGER IS NOT APPROPRIATELY EXPRESSED?

- Anger may be turned inward and forgotten, leading to ulcers, depression, muscle tension, headaches, negative thoughts.

- Anger may "leak out" in indirect ways like accidents, mistakes, poor communication, forgetfulness, word blocks, procrastination, withdrawal, tardiness, and general inefficiency.

8. **PUT YOUR ENERGY INTO CONFIDENCE.** Do not be your own worst enemy. This is a dog-eat-dog world, but it is not the world you are weary of when you become a victim with low self-esteem. *Happiness or misery is a choice you make. The most difficult thing people have to learn is that you can not go around blaming the world for your unhappiness. IF YOU ARE UNHAPPY – IT IS YOUR CHOICE.* People feel victimized because they collapse under the weight of their negative thoughts. It is not stress that is driving you crazy. It is your *response* to stress that makes the difference between *burnout* and *peak performance.*

Accept reality and concentrate on the lessons to be learned. If you give up on yourself, your immune system will too, and you will get sick! Do not waste energy scaring yourself to death with your own negative mental picture. Deal with the reality of today and use your energy to improve *today*. If you interrupt your present negative state, you can alter the outcome of what happens in your life 100% of the time. The situation may stay the same… it is your **ATTITUDE** about it that changes.

> *"THE ENERGY DECLINE IN OLD AGE IS LARGELY THE RESULT OF PEOPLE "EXPECTING TO DECLINE"; THEY HAVE IMPLANTED A SELF-DEFEATING INTENTION IN THE FORM OF A STRONG BELIEF … AND THE MIND/BODY CONNECTION AUTOMATICALLY CARRIES OUT THIS INTENTION."*

- Deepak Chopra

9. **BE ROMANTIC.** Romance is a passionate commitment to happiness. It keeps you from living automatically, and is a right-brain fantasy emotion. Being too romantic is too right-brain. Too unromantic is too left-brain logical. We need BALANCE for enjoyment of life, and protection of health.

    Being romantic is a lot more than being in love with a person; you can be in love with life. Without loving ourselves or our world, we desperately seek out lust for satisfaction … only to find something very important is missing. That frustration makes us angry with ourselves, our world, and the people in it.

10. **GET IN TOUCH WITH THE STATE OF YOUR PHYSICAL HEALTH.** The best mental and emotional suggestions for personal development will fall short of success, if you are sick and tired of being sick and tired. *So, if you do not want to get that way, read on…*

BREAKTHROUGH

I was surrounded by dark walls
    without windows.
The door was closed.
My eyes were open but I could not see.
My mind was closed.
My heart raced with fear and insecurity.
My life was closed.
I cried a lot.

The walls are down now.
The light nearly blinds me.
Possibilities are endless.
Frustrations will cease
    with this feeling of peace.
I have forgotten the dark room.
My life is a fresh bloom.
Excitement
Passion
Joy and fun
Look out world ... here I come!

After a personal growth seminar, about two o'clock in the morning, I was overwhelmed with inspiration. I wrote "Breakthrough" about how I felt. My physical health improved rapidly with my new positive mental and emotional energy.

[] [] [] [] [] []

Now that you have finished the chapter, you may be thinking that the information sounds good on paper, but you wonder if it really works. Believe me, it works ... **and keeps working if that is your choice.** Just like you decided to read this chapter, you can choose to make decisions that further your personal growth, and add quality to life.

Most people have a conscious mind that *minimizes* the driving force behind their thoughts and actions. **An excellent way to get past the blockage is to write out your thoughts.** When you read your own words you are often surprised about how you feel. Being able to reread your thoughts can open up doors that may have been closed for years.

Many people lose their identity during life's struggle. The most rewarding event in your whole life might be finding inner peace with who you are. That means you feel comfortable with your **spiritual** connection, feel **mentally** in control of your today, feel **emotionally** comfortable that you are having your basic needs met, and make choices that allow your **physical** body to work at optimum performance.

I encourage you to give yourself permission to be honest as you write out how you feel. Write about your positive thoughts. Also write about how you feel if you cannot relate to a thought or situation. If you do not take the time to understand yourself, how can you expect anyone else to understand you?

GUIDELINES... NOW GO FOR IT!

1. List activities you could enjoy that allow you to *participate* in life instead of observing. List the ones you plan to look into *now, and what you have to do to get involved!*

    "A CLEAR INTENTION TO REMAIN ACTIVE PRODUCES THE BODY CHEMISTRY THAT ALLOWS US TO REMAIN VIGOROUS AS WE AGE. WHEREVER "THOUGHT" GOES, A CHEMICAL GOES WITH IT. DISTRESSED MENTAL STATES GET CONVERTED INTO THE BIOCHEMICALS THAT CREATE DISEASE."

    - Deepak Chopra

2. List positive words that can encourage you. Affirm them by repeating them as often as you can.

3. List what is not working for you. What payoffs are you getting? Remember, a pay-off means something in your subconscious is getting satisfied.

4. List your mindtraps, why you have them, and how they prevent you **from dealing with your life in a positive way. Remember,** a mindtrap is the way you REACT today to a suppressed fear, or negative experience.

5. Determine your current personality group. Determine the personality group of your family members, co-workers, and friends. Assess how this information can improve these relationships.

6. State your goals, how you are stuck, and how you can improve your determination. Revise your goals to realistic levels.

7. List your fears (i.e. I am not attractive) and then how each fear controls you (i.e. striving for compliments). Decide on some positive affirmations you can repeat often each day. Read the Bach Flower Remedy list again. Even without the remedies you can state the affirmations.

8. Connect with your spiritual self, and listen to your inner voice for Guidance ... a Higher Power may be talking to you. Be willing to take a risk, if you get a strong vibe to stretch yourself.

9. Write your own winning-in-life statement. WHAT DO YOU WANT? *Find out what turns your lights on.* You know when you have inner glow ... a feeling of self-esteem rooted so deep that nothing can make you doubt yourself. Have a statement on paper to read ... read again ... and read again throughout your life. This is my winning-in-life statement, printed on bright pink paper, exactly as I wrote it 18 years ago:

WINNING IN LIFE

WINNING in life to me is:
LIVING in my center.
BEING all I am each day.
REMEMBERING my bond is with the simple life,
I love my part in the balance of nature.
ACKNOWLEDGING I am childlike
And a leader … LIVING in the moment.
In my intimate relationship,
REMEMBERING I am loving, caring, and a companion,
… secure in myself.
ALLOWING openness,
SHARING my knowledge and compassion are my gifts to the
world,
And KNOWING I am honest and tranquil.
My mind and body CELEBRATE my confidence and well being
as I sparkle from within.
I feel beautiful.
I am the source of magic in my life and the world around me.
I AM FORGIVING, CARING OF OTHERS,
AND WORTHY OF LOVE.

Dori C. Luneski
November 20, 1984

This poem by an unknown author fits an aphorism… a statement
of truth:

There is no defeat in life
Save from within,
Unless you're beaten there
You're bound to win.

10. Acknowledge both positive and negative responses you get
from others. Apply what you have learned to improve your
own behavior, or increase your self-confidence.

10. Prioritize your problems, and decide on a plan to accept or resolve them. Balance all that left brain work with some fun, a smile, or a laugh EVERY DAY!

11. Start each day with a positive attitude. *Today* is the only day that can make a difference in your life!

> *"LET YOUR ENTHUSIASM RADIATE IN YOUR VOICE, YOUR ACTIONS, YOUR FACIAL EXPRESSIONS, YOUR PERSONALITY, THE WORDS YOU USE, AND THE THOUGHTS YOU THINK! NOTHING GREAT WAS EVER ACHIEVED WITHOUT ENTHUSIASM."*
>
> - Ralph Waldo Emerson

I wrote this one beautiful morning:

> **Good morning world!**
> **The sun shines even through the rain.**
> **Drops glisten on my windowpane.**
> **I smile and let the day begin.**

BY NOW YOU SHOULD HAVE THE IDEA THAT ...

> ***"LIFE IS A DARING ADVENTURE, OR IT IS NOTHING."***
>
> - Helen Keller

So smile ...

you are just starting your daring adventure!

    To make your daring adventure healthier ... read on to achieve optimum levels of *physical* health. This requires you to evaluate your "intention" to produce results. In the equation "INTENTION + MECHANICS = RESULTS" consider what part of 100% do you give to "INTENTIONS" and what part of 100% do you give to "MECHANICS" which is the choice of how you do something. No combination is correct unless you gave 100% to "INTENTION" and 0% to "MECHANICS". You can always change the *way* you do something if your *intention* to get it done is high enough.

IF YOUR INTENTION TO TAKE RESPONSIBILITY FOR YOUR "WELLNESS" IS 100%... NOW READ ON FOR THE MECHANICS OF HOW TO DO THAT.

CHAPTER 2

NUTRITION

There is a plaque that says, "YOUR HEALTH IS TOO IMPORTANT TO PLACE IN THE HANDS OF YOUR DOCTOR."

Nutrition is not the whole health story, but it is something for which there is no substitute. The several pounds of nutrients you put into your mouth each day are the biggest single determinants of your health.

Americans started the most costly health changes in history when they began living on refined foods, changing from the general use of herbs to synthetic drugs, and decreasing *pure* water intake for less hydrating, and less healthy liquids. Americans cling to the hope that medical science will discover drugs and treatments that will allow them to eat, drink, and be merry, while still maintaining good health. THIS HAS BEEN A MYTH FOR YEARS!

Modern health theories have proven to be a disaster to our general health! With infections, epidemics, and injuries being managed very well by modern medicine, children and young adults are now suffering from chronic poor health, cancer and other diseases. SOMETHING IS OBVIOUSLY VERY WRONG!!! In an experiment by Frances Pottenger, Jr., M.D. on the effects of diet on lab animals, he concluded that only one generation of processed food produced health changes.

Americans eat far from a balanced diet. Ask any schoolteacher if they believe diet does not affect mind, and mood. If acknowledged, that could be a powerful beginning to improve our ailing education system. Children with the most refined, junky, and adulterated diets are the ones most likely to goof off, flunk, get sick, or be inconsistent in motivation. More than ever before, children need natural whole food, healthy snacks, and pure water.

*Most people do not worry about their **total** health if they have a cavity. A CAVITY IS BODY LANGUAGE THAT THE **BODY** IS NOT HEALTHY ... NOT JUST THE TOOTH!*

Our health statistics are a national disaster. That is partly due to the fact that healthy diets are a joke. We are the only country in the world where being health conscious makes you a "health nut." One elderly gentleman in my nutrition class defined healthy food by saying, *"If it tastes good, spit it out."* Food taste is a matter of habit; some cultures drink animal blood. You love heavily sugared desserts, fat-marbled meats, and chemical-laden goodies because these are the foods our generation has been taught to enjoy. Habits can be just as easily good, as bad. If you can *retrain* your taste to enjoy the foods that will *build* health and not destroy it, you are now open to believe that you *will* enjoy the food that provides good nutrition.

Americans are too often motivated by taste appeal, rather than food that we know will improve or maintain our health. We tend not to make *DAILY* dietary choices that protect our *FUTURE HEALTH*. Too many people are indifferent to life. They may not want to die, but when asked about their poor *choices* say, "You have to die sometime." Without a plan and future goal, people too often live only for immediate pleasures. With our abundance of food we think we are well fed today ... or, we will eat better tomorrow. Too often tomorrow is the same fast-paced rat race we had yesterday. It is not the quantities we consume, but our *choices* of what we eat that is one reason for nutritional deficiencies in our country today.

We are a well fed, malnourished society, and health statistics agree. According to the *Illustrated Book of World Rankings* published in 1997, the life expectancy for women in the United States ranks 26th among 187 nations; for men it is 33rd; for infant mortality we are in 25th place. We are a world leader in many areas, yet our national health statistics are shocking. We have epidemic numbers of cancer, heart disease, high blood pressure, osteoporosis, multiple sclerosis, diabetes, and other diseases that cripple children and adults alike. We have a society dealing with every symptom in the book from acne to severe depression, from general pain and fatigue to crisis situations that affects health and financial stability. We eat huge amounts of greasy, salty or sugary *fast food*; highly refined and processed food; and we poison our bodies with caffeine, alcohol, additives and chemicals. Then, we call it bad luck or blame it on heredity when we reach a state of continuous poor health.

Our poor eating habits have cost us dearly. Health care expenses are rapidly escalating. It is now difficult or impossible for many people to afford needed medical attention. The average person lives with *chronic* symptoms that reduces the quality of life. Most people only go for medical attention when symptoms become unbearable, or life threatening. To turn current health trends around, we must make dietary and lifestyle changes to practice **prevention of disease and not wait until we have to treat disease!** Never before has there been a greater need for the practice of *"NEWTRITION"* than today!

[] [] [] [] []

THE VILLAINS

You EARN your good health by your willingness to make proper food selections, and eliminate unhealthy habits. If you wish to improve or protect your health you need to *stop* buying food products that can *contribute to illness*. For economy you may need to clean up what you have already purchased. You can choose to make better choices when you shop next time. *Here are some guidelines for what to avoid in your future grocery shopping:*

1. WHITE SUGAR AND EVERYTHING MADE WITH IT:

This does not mean you cannot have your birthday cake, or an occasional social dessert. You make or break your health at home, and it is there that you should consume the kind of food that is health building.

Your body needs protein, fat, carbohydrates, vitamins and minerals. Sugar contributes only carbohydrates. Because it goes quickly into the bloodstream raising the blood sugar level and satisfying your appetite, it crowds out your desire to eat other foods *that would provide the other nutrition you need.* Raising your blood sugar may be important following heavy exercise or work, but too many people sustain high blood sugar levels when it is not required for normal body function.

The whiplash rise and fall in blood sugar on a regular basis over-stresses your immune system. Sugar is highly addictive and is the third major component of the American diet, after meat and milk. The top dietary choices are often consumed excessively, and can produce many health problems. It is easier to become addicted to sugar than heroin because of accessibility, cost, and social acceptance.

Do not feel you can improve your health by substituting so called healthier sugars. There is no such thing as a guilt-free goody. Excess sugar not needed for normal body function, whether an apple or a candy bar, feeds undesirable intestinal organisms like Candida yeast or parasites. *THE CURE FOR ALL DISEASES* or *THE CURE FOR ALL CANCERS* by Hulda Clark, discusses how parasites can cause any disease in the body. I highly recommend you purchase at least one book on Candida yeast, and one book on parasites for your "wellness" library!

Sugars other than white refined sugar that may fool you into thinking they are healthier include:

- **BROWN SUGAR:** This is white refined sugar with a little molasses added. At least use dark brown sugar for a few more nutrients, but do not kid yourself it improves your health.

- **TURBINADO:** This is the last stage before white sugar, and is minimally better for you. At best it has fewer chemicals. A cookie jar full of turbinado cookies will feed just as many Candida yeast and parasites as white sugar cookies.

- **FRUCTOSE:** Commercially it is mostly derived from corn. One good quality of fructose is that it does not stress the digestive system like white sugar, since it is already a monosaccharide (simple sugar). Unfortunately, it is a chemically refined sugar. Consumed in excess, fructose can increase absorption of triglycerides. Whenever a greater quantity of carbohydrates enter the body than can be immediately used for energy or stored in the liver, the excess is converted to fatty acids called triglycerides. Problems with high triglyceride levels are discussed in the Internal Energy chapter. *For health reasons, you should limit your fructose, but this non-bake cookie recipe can be an occasional treat:*

  In a saucepan mix 1 cup fructose sugar, ¼ cup unsweetened cocoa, ½ cup soy or rice milk, 1 stick hormone and antibiotic free butter, and bring to a full rolling boil. Boil one minute then remove from heat. Quickly add 3 cups quick-cooking oatmeal, ½ rounded cup of smooth or chunky peanut butter without hydrogenated oils or sugar added, and 1 teaspoon vanilla. Spread out on a cookie sheet and place in the refrigerator to cool. Cut into squares; layer separated by foil or wax paper in a tightly sealed container. Refrigerate, and take out "one" for an occasional treat. Unbelievably simple and delicious. Any nut butter like almond, and added chopped almonds can be substituted.

- **SUCANAT:** This sugar is naturally dried cane juice made from organically grown sugar cane with the entire natural vitamins and minerals. Sucanat is not chemically refined, but some chemicals are needed in the processing. This is nutritionally better, but still needs to be in moderation. *Remember, Candida yeast and parasites do not care how "natural" the sugar is, because all sugar breaks down to the simple sugar they need for food!.*

61

- **ARTIFICIAL SWEETENERS:** The body is not fooled, and gets "quick" sugar one way or another. People using artificial sweeteners often consume too much fruit, fruit juices, refined grains, and sugary treats. Artificial sweeteners are still being studied. Some "safe" choices became carcinogenic concerns, or accumulate in cells and damage protein and DNA. Now the choices are 100 percent safe ... until new shocking tests are revealed. *We are human guinea pigs for research.*

2. TOBACCO

Few people know.how tobacco is cured. Our forefathers used natural drying methods, and did not add anything to the tobacco. Many European brands are still using natural drying methods today. Modern American tobacco can be sugar cured. People who smoke are generally unaware of the doubly addictive properties of **both** sugar and tobacco.

Very often in our society, a person who stops smoking increases consumption of candy bars, gum and other sweets in greater quantities than before. They not only have to struggle with the tobacco withdrawal, but they may gain weight as well. The sugar in tobacco keeps the blood sugar up, so a person may not eat as much as they should for healthy body function. In a frantic effort for the body to get the nutrition it needs, a person may suddenly want something to eat. Those choices are too often processed quick foods, not healthy foods.

When you stop smoking, stop eating *ALL REFINED SUGAR, NATURAL SUGAR, AND FRUIT* for one month minimum. This allows your body to fight off the allergic hold the sugar had on your system. You'll soon find your sweet cravings less strong. Gradually, you may add tiny amounts of natural sugars and fresh fruit back into your diet, but no refined sugar except for an occasional social situation.

You did not start smoking because it stinks, costs a lot, and can cause serious health problems. So, you will not likely stop for those reasons. Find out the reasons you are blocking or running from life. Deal with it, work through it, and you will likely **want** to make better health choices. Refer to "quit smoking" techniques on page 285.

3. TOO MUCH REFINED SALT

Salt is big business! Businesses increase their profit by playing on human addictions to substances like refined salt and refined sugar. Be selective! Select unprocessed foods that do not contain refined ingredients. When you prepare meals from scratch you can add healthier seasalt, and other nutritious ingredients.

Organic sodium is a nutrient vital to life. Refined salt (pure sodium chloride) has been heated, and is missing the buffering minerals that make salt a balanced food. This imbalanced product creates health problems; unrefined solar or sun-evaporated sea salt is not imbalanced. Healthy solar sea salt is not your enemy like refined salt. A salt free diet should not eliminate whole alive foods like solar sea salt. *Solar salt is nature's salt ... and is good for you in moderation!* Healthy salt, which is processed only by sun and wind, has a moisture content that contains trace elements essential for health. When the moisture is removed, over seventy valuable trace minerals are lost, and what remains is only sodium chloride ... an enemy to good health. You get the unhealthy sodium in many ways besides in table salt, such as sodium benzoate, sodium nitrate, sodium nitrite, monosodium glutamate, and sodium in city water, and water softeners.

4. ALL CAFFEINE EXCEPT GREEN TEA

Caffeine is a member of the same addictive alkaloid group of chemicals as morphine, nicotine, cocaine, and purines in meat. People addicted to caffeine may also have other addictions like smoking, crave refined sugar, and eat lots of red meat. Stress, addictions, and poor dietary choices generally produce a too acid system.

Our caffeine intake is the largest in the world. Besides coffee, caffeine (or a similar effect) is found in tea, soft drinks, chocolate, and stimulant drugs. The stimulation from caffeine causes the adrenal glands to release hormones that raise the pulse. This signals the liver to release stored sugar; when that sugar reaches the blood it is as much a challenge for the pancreas as consumed sweets. This process robs vitamins, minerals and energy from normal body functions ... which gives you even more body stress. *High caffeine use can ...*

- exhaust the pancreas; can contribute to hypoglycemia or diabetes.

- irritate stomach and intestines.

- imbalance body pH.

- support Candida yeast and parasites overgrowth; worse if consumed with sugar.

- stimulate the central nervous system, and contribute to insomnia, nervousness, and fatigue.

- stimulate the heart, and may be a cause of pulse irregularities.

- increase urination and cause dehydration, and loss of nutrients.

- be a suspect in breast lumps and birth defects.

- contain many chemicals that are used in growing, processing and shipping of caffeine products.

* *One exception is Green Tea, which may be one of the most potent disease preventing substance known. Green Tea can have anti-bacterial, anti-viral, anti-fungal, immune stimulating, anti cancer and circulatory*

benefits. For the same 20% caffeine as in decaffeinated coffee, Green Tea can provide many health benefits. It is available in both plain, and naturally flavored fruit teas; in capsules (should be vegicaps); also decaffeinated. Substituting Green Tea is generally very helpful to prevent headache withdrawal symptoms when you attempt to stop caffeine addictions like coffee, regular tea, or caffeine containing carbonated drinks.

Commercial concerns have fooled the public into thinking that decaffeinated coffee is a healthful substitute. The chemicals first used to decaffeinate coffee were proven to be carcinogenic. Now, different processes are being used ... assumed to be 100 percent safe, until perhaps they are later found to be carcinogenic! If you drink decaffeinated coffee on a regular basis, you could be surprised someday that a product you trusted is not safe at all. Do you want to let unproven modern methods determine the quality of your life? There is usually a hidden problem with every modern-day food and drug *breakthrough.* Forgetting *"new and improved"* is a good place to start. *The next time you are sitting in a doctor's office, and are sick and tired of being sick and tired, decide if any unhealthy dietary choices are worth it.*

Getting back to basics may be your best defense against poor health. If you insist on drinking an occasional social or morning cup of coffee, purchase unfumigated, unsprayed organic coffee beans from a health food store, and store in the freezer. Grind only enough to consume one cup a day. Ground coffee must be kept in the freezer, because the oils quickly turn rancid. If you drink coffee for an energy lift, you will be better off finding the cause of your fatigue. If you are drinking coffee because you like it, you should look for a healthier substitute like herbal tea, grain coffee substitutes, Green Tea, hot lemon water, blackstrap molasses in hot water, *or learn to like plain water.* If all other reasoning fails, at least remember MODERATION, and for every cup of liquid containing caffeine, drink an extra glass of filtered water.

5. WHITE FLOUR AND EVERYTHING MADE WITH IT

Commercial products are geared more towards profit than nutrition. White flour lasts longer. It is lighter in baking, so those products appeal to our modern taste. White flour will not spoil, will not draw bugs and rodents like whole grain flour, and is supposedly "enriched" for your health. It looks like the bugs and rodents are more selective than we are! In refining, about 28 nutrients are removed, and about six synthetic nutrients added. *THIS CAN HARDLY BE CALLED* **ENRICHED**. White flour is a simple sugar; whole grains are complex carbohydrates that break down slowly to simple sugars.

White flour is not the *staff of life*. Its empty calories quickly convert to energy, but the body is still waiting for nutrients needed for healthy elimination, and cellular function.

Our low-fiber, refined diet acts like glue in the intestines. Modern machinery has taken the outer layer off the grain and removed the germ. Without the germ, flour is a dead food. LIVE FOOD IS FOR LIVE PEOPLE ... IF MOLD WILL NOT GROW ON IT, NEITHER WILL YOU! DO NOT MESS WITH MOTHER NATURE!!! Our modern *"new and improved"* foods are creating a sick and diseased society.

When you read labels look for *whole* wheat as the first word. Commercial labeling is tricky; wheat flour is not whole wheat. Stone ground whole wheat has higher protein than other processes. Bakery products sold in health food stores will generally have far less chemicals than commercial products, but may still contain refined flour. Vegetable pasta such as beet or spinach is still refined flour.

6. ALCOHOL - REMEMBER MODERATION

Moderation is as important with alcohol as it is with coffee. An occasional favorite drink may not be a major health issue if you do not feel bad after you drink it, or feel worse the next morning. How you interpret the words "occasional" or "moderation" could be an important factor. Living the "good life" is not so good when you get sick.

Dealing with emotional issues by strengthening your self confidence and feeling of security, will always be a more healthful approach than escape through alcohol. One drink may not be an overwhelming hazard to your health; but, if you NEED that drink to relax, then you are using alcohol in a harmful way. You should understand whether you are controlling the alcohol, or the alcohol is controlling you. *The negative effects of daily alcohol consumption are many:*

- **Changes the body's ability to metabolize zinc,** needed to make many hormones and enzymes in the body.

- **Expands the cells of the intestine** so alcohol and food can be absorbed into the bloodstream without complete digestion. This can produce intestinal and liver stress called "Leaky Gut Syndrome" (discussed in the Elimination chapter). This problem can be the basis for many other symptoms. *ALCOHOL CONSUMED WITH A MEAL PRODUCES A MUCH GREATER RISK OF ALLERGIC REACTIONS.*

- **Supports emotional crutches:**

  * not dealing with low self-esteem.

  * not working on poor health that produces symptoms of low blood sugar.

  * not being aware that cravings may be due to allergic withdrawal to grains, sugar, yeast, and certain fruits.

  * not being aware of the dietary demands needed to support Candida yeast and/or parasite overgrowth.

- **Stresses the hardest working organ of your body ... your liver.** The reasons to "love your liver" are discussed in the Digestion chapter.

- **Affects the body the same as any simple sugar.** If you are drinking alcohol with sweets, you are giving your body a doubly harmful effect.

7. ALL PROCESSED AND REFINED FOODS

IF IT IS *NEW AND IMPROVED*, FORGET IT! Only natural, unprocessed food can give you a full quota of vitamins and minerals in a state that your body can effectively use.

People can be fooled nutritionally. Soil tests show dramatic differences in mineral content of our agricultural lands. Chemical fertilizers do not replace many of the nutrients taken from the land by continuous cropping. Some foods are picked green and gas ripened. *This story about canned peas gives you an example of what nutrition you are not getting:*

> *Plants cannot take up nutrients that are not available in the soil, so a crop of peas grown commercially today will not have the same nutritional quality as peas grown a generation ago. Further nutrients are lost in transportation and washing. When the peas are canned, minerals are again lost in the water and some vitamins are affected in various degrees. Heat destroys **all** enzymes to assist in digestion, so now your body must do all the work. Storage and distribution practices vary, but the canned peas could be several years old when you decide to cook them for dinner. Then you boil the peas and throw the mineral-rich water down the drain, so your unhealthy hydrogenated margarine will stick to them. After the farmer, the packer, the grocer, and you have done your best to eliminate every vestige of nutrition from those peas, you take comfort in having eaten your vegetable for dinner!*

We must stop kidding ourselves that the food we put into our mouths contains all the nutrients we see listed in the food charts. Commercial farming, processing, refining, storage, additives, and cooking all contribute to nutritionally deficient meals. JUST BECAUSE YOU ARE NOT HUNGRY DOES NOT MEAN

YOUR CELLS ARE WELL FED! Since you live or die on a cellular level, for good health you must eat food that gives you a *fighting chance* to be healthy. Given the increase stress levels from social, family, career, environmental and chemical changes, we can no longer get what we need from the food we eat. HIGH QUALITY **NATURAL FOOD** SUPPLEMENTATION IS CRITICAL TO SURVIVE IN OUR MODERN TIMES!

Fresh is always best, as long as the fresh is not old and wilted. Dried is second best, because low heat does not destroy enzymes and nutrients like high heat. Mold may be a problem in dried food if you are mold sensitive. Frozen food is next, but should be purchased in a health food store; commercial brands may contain EDTA to preserve freshness that can bind some nutrients, and reduce absorption. Canned food is least nutritious; if eaten, do not through away the liquid that contains valuable minerals. If you have an excess of mineral-rich produce from your organic garden, you may choose to can that produce, but you will preserve more food value if you dry or freeze.

8. EXCESSIVE AMOUNTS OF PROTEIN

Americans eat too much animal protein. The recommended amount of protein varies greatly depending on age, activity, exercise and general health. In spite of our medical research and technological advantages, Americans are a disease-ridden population. The average consumption of protein in this country, plus high protein weight loss diets, may double or triple the daily needs ... *and that spells ill health in many ways:*

- **Imbalances the B vitamins**, since large amounts of B6 and B3 are needed to metabolize protein.

- **Production of ammonia**, (dangerous by-product of animal protein metabolism), found to be a carcinogenic. There is a high rate of colon and rectal cancer in our society obsessed with meat.

69

- **Impairment of calcium absorption** due to high levels of phosphorus in red meat that can cause calcium loss. That loss may lead to calcium deficiency related diseases such as osteoporosis, osteoarthritis, dental disease, and allergies. In Japan, osteoporosis is low because their diet is low in protein. Calcium balance is determined not only by the amount of calcium you eat, but also by the amount of protein. Excess protein creates acid waste that is neutralized by calcium in amounts that can cause calcium depletion.

- **Increased rise in kidney failure** because the kidneys are overstressed excreting breakdown products.

- **Imbalance of acid/alkaline pH** that can cause cravings for acid foods and create addictions to grains, caffeine, carbonated drinks, sugar, alcohol, tobacco, and drugs. An imbalanced pH discussed in the Digestion Chapter, causes people to flock to the drugstore for a barrage of *"new and improved"* digestive and elimination aids.

- **Deficiency of Vitamin A** needed to connect amino acids into protein chains.

- **Elevates triglyceride levels** when people eat more protein than needed. A large share of *excess* protein is stored as fat; a high triglyceride level can be caused by excess stored protein or carbohydrates.

The body does not store protein as it does fat and carbohydrates, so the food companies have made Americans afraid of getting too little dietary protein. Red meat is a social issue; the more money you make, the more you can afford to eat red meat! Beans are sometimes associated with poverty, and poor quality incomplete protein. Actually incomplete proteins eaten the *SAME DAY* can *CREATE* complete proteins, because we have internal reserves of amino acids to fill in as needed.

70

Of the 22 amino acids required to build a complete protein, nine cannot be formed by the body, but must be consumed in the diet. No matter what the "eat more meat" advertising tells you, a mixture of animal *AND* vegetable proteins is used most efficiently by the body. Animal protein does not have to be red meat (beef, buffalo, lamb, pork or venison). Hormone and antibiotic-free chicken or turkey, organic eggs, fresh fish and seafood are all easier to digest. Those foods supply the type of needed brain phosphorus that is different than the phosphorus found in vegetables. The loss of this *form* of phosphorus is one reason why intellectually driven vegetarians often suffer with fatigue. They are overworking the brain, but not providing what nutrients it needs.

Red meat is very hard to digest and puts considerable stress on the liver. Consume red meat in small amounts, not more than twice a week, and always hormone and antibiotic-free. Avoid high-fat, processed, and commercial lunchmeats. *Do not be fooled with trick advertising:*

> *95 percent fat free refers to "weight" of the fat left, and not calories. In 2 percent milk there are five grams of fat and 140 calories per serving. To figure out how many calories in 2 percent milk come from fat, multiply five by nine to convert grams to calories; divide that by total number of calories and you get 45 divided by 140 = 32 percent of the calories come from fat; 2 percent sounds better than 32 percent fat. KEEP TOTAL FAT INTAKE AT OR BELOW 20-25 PERCENT OF CALORIES, AND SATURATED FAT AT 7 PERCENT OF CALORIES OR LESS FOR EACH FOOD ITEM.*

SOME PROTEIN FACTS WORTH KNOWING:

- *Beef eye round is the part of the beef lowest in fat and cholesterol. It is still hard to digest, is mucus forming, and may produce unwanted allergic reactions you do not realize are from the beef. If you eat beef sparingly,* ***always*** *buy hormone and antibiotic-free.*

71

- *Veal commercially grown should be boycotted, because of the outrageous animal cruelty to produce tender meat, and callous disregard for human health as the pale meat of veal comes from animals low in iron.*

- *Lamb is lower in fat because the fat is marbled on the outside and easier to remove. Beef is higher in fat because it is marbled throughout the meat. Non-organic lamb purchased in regular grocery stores contains less hormones and antibiotics than other red meats.*

- *Fish should be rotated to protect against any local pollution problems. Even fresh fish can be shockingly contaminated by bacteria. Either dip in 3% food-grade hydrogen peroxide (as well as meat and fowl), then rinse in water, and wipe dry; or wash well under full pressure faucet water, and wipe dry.*

- *Animal products are full of antibiotics that imbalance intestinal flora. The influence of hormones given to animals including pork, contributing to our poor health statistics is still being researched. There are some **horror stories** about the quality used for some commercial products like soup, or cut-up meat products. Purchase organic animal products; or obtain from small market owners dealing with farmers direct, so they know how the animal was raised.*

9. CHEMICAL FOOD ADDITIVES

IF YOU CAN'T PRONOUNCE IT, DON'T EAT IT! I can pronounce *apple*. Butylated hydrexyanisole, tertiary butylhydroquinone are chemicals used in some salad dressings, that do not sound like words said around the old country wood stove.

It is quite a surprise when you read lists of ingredients on the packages of highly processed foods in your grocery store. They

72

look like shopping lists for chemists! I live simply ... back to basics. I have absolute standards for the food I purchase for my home. When I go to a restaurant, I order sensibly, or even indulge occasionally; the rule is, YOU MAKE OR BREAK YOUR HEALTH AT HOME. I am never tempted to purchase products that contain preservatives, artificial coloring or flavoring, nitrates or nitrites, monosodium glutamate, refined sugar or flour, EDTA, or other additives. We are told these chemicals are perfectly safe, but current health statistics suggest something is very wrong. *Consumers need to continue demanding healthier food! The products you choose to purchase have tremendous power in what the industry will produce in the future!!!*

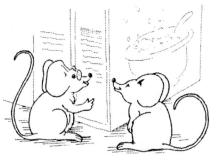

We're not touchin' any of this stuff
until we find something NUTRITIOUS!

One organization that deserves credit for studying the effects of chemicals in our diet is the Feingold Association. Their research has shown a connection between hyperactivity in children and consumption of food additives and sugar. Many hyperactive children turn into irritable, nervous adults. The Feingold information can help all ages. Check your telephone book for the local association number.

Eat simple unprocessed, non-chemical whole foods in their natural, uncomplicated form. Chemicals have only been in existence since World War II. Considering the appalling health of the general population, it is hard to believe our bodies can adjust so quickly to so many invasive changes. Truth is ... it has not adjusted! But, disease in this country is politically controlled, and is BIG BUSINESS!

10. SATURATED FAT AND HYDROGENATED OILS

FATS FALL INTO THREE CATEGORIES:

- Highest in saturated fats are red meat, coconut and palm oils, and lard; these harden at room temperature.

- Highest in monounsaturated fats are flaxseed, olive, almond, avocado, and peanut oils; these are liquid at room temperature.

- Highest in polyunsaturated fats are safflower, sunflower, soy and corn oils; also liquid at room temperature.

Deciding what oil to use should be based on the oil's ability to change to trans-fatty acid formation. Trans-fatty acids are unnatural to the body and bad for your health. Monounsaturated fats are not subject to as much trans-fatty acid formation, so oils high in monounsaturated fats are the current health trend. Canola oil is hybridized rapeseed, and is a major crop in Canada (Can-ola). Website information from Canadian companies may not be the best source of information about standards of processing of this controversial oil.

Polyunsaturated oils first became popular because of their ability to lower serum cholesterol. They are nutritious and beneficial when fresh, but are especially subject to attack by oxygen. Outside your body this means oil becomes rancid; inside the body it undergoes a similar change forming free radicals that may lead to disease. Another problem is polyunsaturated fats also reduce HDL levels, the good cholesterol. Monounsaturated oils lower LDL cholesterol too, but have a neutral effect on HDL cholesterol.

When Americans started to understand the relationship between fats and health, the commercial food industries had to do something fast. They could not protect their investment if chosen oils turned rancid. They had to "invent" an oil that would act like a saturated fat, but the label could read *no saturated fat*. In their infinite wisdom they came up with hydrogenated oils. Do not be fooled by modern science. Remember, IF IT IS NEW AND IMPROVED, MANUFACTURERS MAY SMILE ALL THE WAY TO THE BANK, BUT IT MAY NOT GOOD FOR YOUR HEALTH!

> ***Unsaturated** fats can be converted into **saturated** fats by a process called **hydrogenation,** so they will not become rancid during frying or while being stored. This process acts like a chemical hair-straightener, turning natural, curved unsaturated fatty acids into straight man-made trans-fatty acids. Hydrogenated oils in margarine, vegetable shortening, and most processed foods and snacks are so destructively altered they are worse for your health than saturated animal fats. Until the government is willing to unchain themselves from the politics of the food industry, facts will continue to be blocked from the consumer.*
>
> *Hydrogenation produces high levels of trans-fatty acids which intensify essential fatty acid deficiencies, and produces "weird prostaglandins." Your health depends on the presence of short-lived cellular hormones (some live only a few seconds) called prostaglandins, to act as chemical catalysts in every activity that goes on in your body every second of your life. Your body does not make prostaglandins. They are made by the breakdown process of the essential fatty acids in foods like whole grains, nuts and seeds, and cold-pressed oils. Refining removes the "life" part of the oil, and all that is left is the fat; refining removes the "life" from the grain.*

Always buy cold-pressed oils and refrigerate, because they have not been refined, and still contain the essential fatty acids needed by your body. IF AN OIL WILL NOT TURN RANCID, IT WILL NOT DO YOU ANY GOOD! Again, new and improved is generally not healthier. **YOU CANNOT IMPROVE ON NATURE!!!**

All vegetable oils are cholesterol-free. Labeling laws have improved, but often the details are overlooked with packaging headlines like *"Made with 100 percent vegetable oil"* or *"No cholesterol."* These products may contain tropical saturated fats or hydrogenated oils. You need to read ALL the package information, and also know how to interpret *if the fancy label really tells you enough*!

11. MILK AND DAIRY PRODUCTS

"Modern" milk is not the same milk your grandparents consumed. Milk may be the perfect food for calves, but it has no right being called a perfect food for humans. Milk is hard to digest; is mucus forming; and may contain hormones, antibiotics, chemicals, drugs, pesticides, and radioactive strontium from the atmosphere. Milk is a political issue … not a nutritional super food! *Milk has been linked to many physical symptoms such as…*

- colic in babies, and intestinal problems in adults.
- diarrhea, and iron deficiency.
- sinus, ear, respiratory symptoms in children and adults.
- headaches.
- chronic joint pains.
- cold extremities.
- auto-immune diseases (examples like Rheumatoid Arthritis, Multiple Sclerosis, Lupus, Diabetes, and some kidney failure).

THERE ARE SOME FACTS ABOUT MILK YOU SHOULD KNOW:

- We are the only mammals on the earth drinking another mammals milk by choice, and regularly drinking it as adults. Goat's milk is better than cow's milk because it is closer to the composition of human milk. It should be the first choice for babies if mother's milk is not available. The casein (protein) in goat's milk could still be an allergy. All mammary milk has casein.

- Our ability to digest milk sugar (lactose) decreases after about age four. Chronic intestinal problems are often linked to the inability to digest milk sugar. Pasteurization inactivates natural digestive enzymes in milk making it hard to digest. The new ultra-pasteurization destroys even more nutrients ... the shelf life is extended, but at what cost to our health?

- It is surprising how apparent it is that cow's milk can produce disease, and yet it is politically protected by the government, buying and stockpiling excess to prevent price fluctuations.

- Dr. Kurt Oster, a cardiologist, believes homogenized milk releases an enzyme called Xanthine Oxidase, that is absorbed through the intestinal wall, circulates in the blood, and is deposited in the blood vessel wall. Here this lethal enzyme may create the beginning of plaque formation and arteriosclerosis. *MILK THE DEADLY POISON* by Robert Cohen discusses this process, and other ways science has destroyed this natural food. Heart attacks are fewer in countries where milk is not homogenized. Milk is first pasteurized, then homogenized (fat broken up under pressure); most milk products are made from homogenized milk. Heat kills Xanthine Oxidase, but after pasteurization 40 percent still remains. Further cooking of milk in recipes would be better in this instance.

- Cow's milk has 1200 milligrams of calcium per quart, human milk has 300 milligrams. Why does an infant on human milk absorb more calcium? Calcium to phosphorus ratio should be 2-1 or more. Too much phosphorus can reduce calcium absorption. Cow's milk ratio is 1.2-1, human milk ratio is better than 2-1.

77

- Then there is the all-American ice cream … not what Grandma used to make. Ice cream manufacturers are not required by law to list the additives. Those same additives may also be used in some household and industrial products, like paint remover, leather cleaner, lice killer, antifreeze and coal tar. Our society is so addicted to fun food, few people associate their life draining symptoms and diseases to their diet. DELICIOUS MAY NOT BE NUTRITIOUS! Check your health food store for healthier ice cream made from soy or rice milk.

[] [] [] [] [] []

THE HEROES

WE ARE A SICK-ORIENTED SOCIETY THAT THINKS WE CAN EAT, DRINK, AND BE MERRY BECAUSE THE MEDICAL PROFESSION WILL SAVE US. THE TRAINING MOST AMERICANS GET ON HEALTH AWARENESS IS LIKE PUTTING OUT A HOUSE FIRE WITH A SQUIRT GUN. WE TREAT OURSELVES FOR PHYSICAL, EMOTIONAL, AND MENTAL SYMPTOMS, AND ESCAPE INTO ADDICTIVE HABITS BECAUSE WE CANNOT HANDLE OUR STRESSFUL WORLD.

Health metamorphosis occurs when the human body gets what it needs to work at optimum performance … the body heals itself. Here are some basic healthy food tips … THINK HEALTH, NOT DISEASE!

"Let nature be your teacher."

- William Wordsworth

1. NATURAL SUGARS

The sweeteners with some nutritional value are sorghum, honey, maple syrup, and blackstrap molasses. Even these sugars should be eaten in small amounts. I talked to one lady who proudly proclaimed that she did not let her son use any refined sugar, and she wondered if a half cup of honey on his cereal was too much! People who are used to consuming large amounts of refined sugar think they are eating better when they consume just as much natural sugar. Having an assortment of cookies, cakes, pies, and sweet breads always on hand keeps you addicted to sweet foods, whether they were made with refined or natural sugar. Learn to reduce your need for sweet taste. Your obsession for sweets is largely from your microorganisms like Candida yeast and parasites demanding their breakfast, lunch, and dinner!

A FEW FACTS ABOUT NATURAL SUGARS YOU SHOULD KNOW:

HONEY *should be raw, unrefined, unfiltered, and unheated.* Honey is high in fructose, which does not need insulin to break it down. Since fructose is already a simple sugar, it is less of a *digestive* strain than refined sugar. Tupelo honey from Florida and Blackbutton Sage honey are both high in fructose compared to other honeys. The cheapest honey is bought on tap. Mild honey is light in color and taste; darker honeys are stronger flavored, and richer in minerals.

There are many excellent books on cooking, eating, and canning with honey. I want to emphasize that occasional "treat" recipes add fun to life. A person who indulges in a special treat occasionally is less likely to need the Bach Flower Remedy ROCK WATER, listed in the Positive Thinking chapter that states "life's pleasures are suffocated under self-imposed disciplines." *I do not routinely make sweet dinner recipes, but the following is a favorite "party" snack that can be enjoyed occasionally, because you eat right most of the time:*

Purchase 12-14 dejointed chicken wings; trim skin as much as possible, pat dry and place in casserole. Mix 1/2 cup honey with 3 tablespoons cornstarch or arrowroot, 1/2 teaspoon ginger, 1/2 cup water, 1/3 cup fresh squeezed lemon juice, 1/4 cup soy sauce. Cook until thickened, pour over wings and bake at 350 degrees for 45 minutes, turning several times. Place on stove top and cook 15 minutes stirring almost constantly to boil down liquid and glaze - ENJOY!

MAPLE SYRUP is between 60 to 65 percent refined sugar sucrose (white sugar is 99 percent sucrose, honey rarely over 3 percent). The rest is water and minerals. Pure maple syrup can contain dangerous amounts of lead, leached from metal buckets with lead solder. Holes drilled in trees are often kept open with paraformaldehyde pellets. This practice is unlawful in Canada so I always buy Canadian maple syrup. Some New England producers avoid it voluntarily, and will provide affidavits to this effect. Some health food stores offer maple syrup on tap, but mold grows if not refrigerated.

BLACKSTRAP MOLASSES is a by-product of the cane sugar industry. Blackstrap is the first stage in cane sugar refining, and should be chosen over other types of molasses. It is an excellent source of the B vitamins, iron, calcium, potassium, and trace minerals. It is 65 to 70 percent sucrose. One tablespoon of blackstrap molasses in a cup of hot water makes a great mineral drink, and is a natural laxative. *I have a favorite bran muffin recipe that uses blackstrap molasses:*

Soak 1 cup bran in 1 cup soy or rice milk (do not pack) for 5 minutes. Add 1 egg, 1/4 cup cold-pressed oil, 2 full tablespoons blackstrap molasses, and beat well. Mix 1 1/2 cups whole wheat flour, 3 teaspoons baking powder, 1/2 level teaspoon sea salt together; stir into the bran mixture. Bake at 400 degrees for 25-30 minutes in 12 oil sprayed muffin cups.

SORGHUM is an edible tropical grass seed that produces a sweet juice. It is 65 to 70 percent sucrose.

STEVIA is natural and *non-caloric*. It is 200 times sweeter than sugar, and safe even for Candida yeast, parasite overgrowth, or diabetes. Check health food stores for non-caloric sweeteners.

2. SUN-EVAPORATED OR SOLAR SEA SALT

The Grain and Salt Society (refer to Resource References) sells an excellent informative book, and totally natural sea salt from the ocean called Celtic Salt. This completely unrefined salt possesses the power to restore wholeness and balance to our body fluids. DO NOT TAKE THIS RECOMMENDATION CASUALLY. HEALTH MEANS INTERNAL BALANCE!!! Celtic Salt is available finely ground for salt shakers. It still contains some moisture, so you may need to tap the salt shaker occasionally to keep the holes open (do not add rice).

Solar or sun-evaporated seasalt is a second choice over the naturally harvested, chemical-free, and perfectly balanced Celtic Sea Salt (both available health food stores). **Some sea salt is too dried, and has lost the trace mineral content; the label must say solar or sun-evaporated, not just sea salt.**

3. WHOLE GRAINS

Whole grains are rich in fiber and nutrients. They are complex carbohydrates, so they break down slowly in the digestive process. Whole grains do not saturate the system with simple sugar like refined sugars, fruits, dairy products, and refined grains.

Grains need to be either cooked or sprouted for best nutritional absorption. Sprouted grains and unleavened bread are good for yeast sensitive people. Grind grains fresh before using, or buy in small amounts and store in the refrigerator. Whole grains products, unlike processed and refined grains, will turn rancid if not stored in the refrigerator or freezer. Your overworked liver will have to deal with the problem. If the good

81

oils are removed to protect against rancidity, the food does not contain the "good stuff" you need for health, *REFINED FOOD IS DEAD FOOD!*

Develop your taste for *ALL* the whole grains, not just wheat. Grains high in gluten (which cause some people to experience stomach distress, other intestinal complaints, or allergic reactions elsewhere in the body) are wheat, oats, rye, barley, and spelt. A non-grain buckwheat has a gluten-like protein. Some buckwheat products are listed as gluten-free. You may need to try for tolerance. You may tolerate buckwheat on a four day rotation. Spelt is a very tolerated grain, even for some gluten sensitive people if consumed in small amounts on a four day rotation. Health food stores have a full range of bakery items made with spelt; they also carry baked goods with less chemicals and sometimes organically grown ingredients. *If your spelt baked goods do not rise, double the baking powder as I did in this Banana Bread recipe:*

> *Preheat over to 350 degrees. Grease an 8½ by 4½ loaf pan (optional: sprinkle poppy seeds on the bottom and sides.) Whisk together 2/3 cup soy or rice milk and 2 teaspoons lemon juice (or 1 teaspoon vinegar), 1/3 cup cold-pressed oil (like canola), 1/3 cup maple syrup, and 1 egg. Sift 2 cups spelt flour with 1 teaspoon sea salt, 1 teaspoon baking soda, and 4 teaspoons baking powder (2 teaspoons if using whole wheat pastry flour.) To the liquid mixture alternately add dry ingredients and 1 cup mashed ripe banana (whip in blender.) Blend in ½ cup of pecans or other nut of choice. This is a moist banana bread and generally needs 1 hour to bake, but test in 50 minutes to see if a knife inserted in the center comes out clean.*

There are other ways to manage meals without the usual bread. Celery, green or red bell peppers, tomatoes, organic potato skins, romaine lettuce leaves, fresh or steamed cabbage, or chinese cabbage leaves can all hold sandwich ingredients.

Spaghetti squash is a great substitute for wheat spaghetti. Boil spaghetti squash in water to cover, for about 40 minutes, depending on size. Split in half and flip out spaghetti-like strands with a fork. Serve with your favorite sauce.

Non-gluten grains are rice, corn, and millet. Rice cakes and corn tortillas are good bread substitutes for the gluten intolerant. Millet is the forgotten grain although it has been used for 1500 years. It is unfortunate its birdseed appearance has prevented its popularity, because it is one of the most nutritious foods known to man, and the most nutritious grain. Millet and cooked carrots may be helpful for diarrhea. *A macrobiotic cooking class taught me how to make millet delicious:*

> *Cook one cup millet in three cups slightly salted water for 20 minutes; drain. Place one inch of water in a steamer. Cover millet with a towel before placing lid on. As it steams, the towel absorbs the moisture so it does not drip into the millet. The millet puffs up like popcorn into a delicious grain.*

Any grain can be an allergic food. If you have any unexplained chronic symptom, and you crave any grain product, you should suspect an allergy to the grain you eat most often.

TO TEST A GRAIN (DAIRY OR ANY FOOD YOU LOVE TO EAT ON A REGULAR BASIS):

> ***COMPLETELY*** *avoid all grains (or other food being tested) for four days. During this period it is not uncommon to have flu-like withdrawal symptoms, or an aggravated version of an existing symptom. Symptoms usually clear by the end of the fourth day.*
>
> *On the fifth day of withdrawal. pick a time that allows at least two free hours, and **at least one hour when you can sit down**. Record how you feel, and record your pulse taken at your wrist (thumb side) for one full minute. Then eat a small portion of the organic food to be tested. Record symptoms and pulse at 20, 40, and 60 minutes after eating. A pulse increase or decrease of eight points, or any change in symptoms, indicates a probable sensitivity. If there are no*

symptoms eat a second portion of the same food and evaluate symptoms in 30 and 60 minutes.

You may be surprised at how a "healthy food" is the cause of your discomfort. Any food you love to eat, and are seldom out of that food, could be the cause of allergic symptoms.

Three favorite whole grain breakfast or brunch recipes are:

- *Oil and heat waffle iron. To 1 cup whole wheat or spelt flour add 1 tablespoon baking powder, ½ rounded teaspoon sea salt, and 2 teaspoons maple syrup. Add 2 egg yolks, 1 cup rice milk, 1/8 cup cold-pressed oil and beat hard for 2 minutes. Fold in 2 beaten egg whites. Bake until steaming stops for a crisp waffle.*

- *French toast made with 4 slices of any whole grain bread: whip 2 organic eggs, add 1/8 cup rice or soy milk, 1 teaspoon cinnamon, 1/4 teaspoon seasalt (adjust cinnamon and seasalt according to taste); brown, and top with Better Butter (recipe in this chapter) and a small amount of pure maple syrup. For a variation taste treat add a whipped banana or blueberries to French Toast, pancakes, or waffles.*

- *Whole wheat pancakes made with whole wheat or spelt flour: separate two organic eggs and whip whites into stiff peaks. Place yolks in a larger bowl and add 1 cup of flour, 1 cup rice or soy milk, 1 tablespoon cold pressed canola oil (or any other cold pressed oil except olive), 2 teaspoons pure maple syrup to help brown, 1/2 teaspoon sea salt, 1 1/2 teaspoons aluminum-free baking powder. Blend all ingredients, and fold in egg whites. May add 1 cup fresh blueberries or other fruit of choice, if desired. Bake on griddle sprayed with oil (I regularly use an olive oil spray for all pan preparation); top with a small amount of pure maple syrup, optional Better Butter ... ENJOY!*

84

4. VEGETABLES

I can almost guarantee you that if you eat lots of raw vegetables, drink at least eight glasses of filtered water daily for a month, eliminate dairy, red meat, refined sugar, refined grains, and caffeine, you'll notice a distinct change in the way you feel. Vegetables are low in carbohydrates, high in vitamins, minerals, enzymes, aid in digestion, assist in keeping the system from becoming too acid, and are the "regenerators" of the body.

Most vegetables should be eaten raw except rhubarb, beans, peas, potatoes, and corn (a grain). Some vegetables like spinach, asparagus, cauliflower, cabbage and broccoli are high in phytates, which if eaten raw *all the time*, can decrease the availability of the nutrients in those foods. They are best steamed, or eaten raw in moderation.

Chopping exposes cut surface to air causing oxidation, which destroys nutrients like Vitamin A, C, B6, thiamine and biotin. Do not prepare cut vegetables ahead of time, purchase food at grocery salad bars, or purchase packaged precut vegetables. A lot of nutrients are concentrated in the outer layer, so scrub instead of peel if organic. If the nonorganic food looks shiny (like apples and cucumbers), they may be covered with a hydrocarbon wax, and should be peeled.

Give your vegetables proper care after you buy them. Bring them straight home, wash them VERY WELL in an organic cleanser, or a fruit and vegetable wash. Refrigerated vegetables in closed glass jars, zip-lock bags, or large plastic containers stay fresh longer than in the vegetable bin. All food begins to lose nutrients as soon as the food is harvested. Fresh fruits and vegetables are especially perishable, so take care to minimize this deterioration.

Microwave ovens are advertised to retain nutrients, but cooking may change the molecular structure adversely. I no longer choose to experiment with my life using modern technology, or "new and improved" products. I am most comfortable going back to basics since *all* the data will take many years to compile, and may still be missing important health statistics. I heat in my microwave, but never cook longer than two minutes. *NEVER* heat water in the microwave in a ceramic cup as it can leach out lead; or drink out of a ceramic cup when the inside of the cup has cracked glaze. *NEVER STAND IN FRONT AND LOOK AT A MICROWAVE OVEN WHEN IT IS RUNNING!!!*

There are many vegetable shredders on the market, and I have purchased most of them. I do not use some I have purchased, because of disappointing results. The one *successful* one I still use is frequently demonstrated in shopping malls. If you see a vegetable shredder demonstration that looks easy, I suggest you purchase one. I also want to suggest another appliance that I use constantly. It is the *small* food processor that you can cut up a little onion, garlic, celery, etc. easily and quickly without using larger appliances. There are a number of brands available in most stores that carry small appliances; some are demonstrated in shopping malls. *These appliances made easy work of many recipes:*

> *Scrub 2 large organic potatoes and remove the eyes. Use any shredder that makes thin home style cuts of the unpeeled potatoes, and very thin medium white onion pieces. In the chopper place 2 large garlic cloves and 3-4 sprigs of parsley. Low heat cook all ingredients in olive oil until home fries are done, about 30 minutes. Season as desired, and add to any meal from breakfast to dinner.*

Steaming (drink mineral-rich liquid left in pan), stir frying, or waterless cooking are best ways to cook vegetables because nutrients are not lost in discarded water. Soup is a good mineral rich food. One appliance everyone should own is an eight quart stainless steel steamer. It can be used as a vegetable streamer, a pasta cooker, and a soup pot.

Cooking in a pressure cooker has been forgotten in recent years. This is a shame because protein, starches and vegetables cook up quickly and taste naturally sweet. Pressure cooking allows you to cook less frequently consumed root vegetables, and time consuming meats and vegetables in usually under 30 minutes. *A delicious dinner (including the liquid) is:*

> *One hormone and antibiotic-free skinned chicken. Add a combination of carrots, onions, cabbage, potatoes, parsnips, or turnips as desired. Salt with sea salt. Water and cooking time is based on the book that comes with the cooker. Very quickly you have a nutritious dinner!*

Learn to be a bean lover! Legumes are high in fiber, protein, many necessary nutrients, low in fat, and provide recipes that keep you from eating so much red meat. Many people avoid them because of their gas-forming properties (indigestible sugars that the body cannot break down). You can buy a digestive product for beans at health food stores if you like beans, but not the side effects. *If you prepare your beans correctly, you may be able to enjoy them without distress:*

> *Soak overnight or 4-6 hours and discard the water. This soaking may be enough to eliminate problems; if not try this next step. Cover with water and bring to a boil; boil one minute and discard that water. The beans can then be boiled in the amount of water that is not completely absorbed. When they are soft, discard the cooking water before using the beans in your favorite recipe. Some people may tolerate omitting the last part, and cook the beans in the finished product, like soup. Cooked beans freeze well; make enough for multiple quick meals. If you freeze plain cooked beans, thaw and add to cold salads.*
>
> *If you cook black-eyed peas, you can freeze them in serving sizes, thaw as desired and toss with cold-pressed mayonnaise and chopped white onions. If you cannot tolerate onions, add any desired vegetable, like tomatoes or cucumber to cooked beans and mayonnaise.*

New vegetables at the family dinner table may meet shocking resistance. When introducing new foods to your family, cook QUIETLY! You do not have to announce that the family spaghetti sauce contains wheat germ. Shock treatment of making a friend's favorite blueberry pie with whole wheat crust and honey is not the place to start teaching healthier eating. At one family meal, I served soup with seaweed in it. My son asked, "What's that green stuff floating around in my soup?" When I explained that it was seaweed, my husband said, "You had to ask?"

Changing the family diet is like breaking ground ... one shovelful at a time. Adjustments of any kind can be a challenge, because our food obsessions in this country make dietary changes a social discomfort.

*Many children and teens have a particularly difficult time suddenly adjusting to a healthier diet, because there is so much peer pressure to consume junk food. Children and teens sometimes refuse to support family changes as a way of getting back for past conflicts. They may be upset with a parent, so there is no way they will make any transition easily. A family compromise that works very well is having the "adults" in the family who make the money to buy the groceries, make a **statement of fact** that they are responsible for buying the groceries that will be eaten **in the home**. This makes a firm statement of "fact" that healthier food choices **will** be purchased. Children and teens can then feel free to meet whatever social standards they consider necessary when they are **out of the home** without parents putting a guilt trip on them.*

If a child or teenager protests unreasonably about the change, the parent should calmly say there are only three choices:

- *They can choose to eat what has been purchased, or prepared.*

- *They can choose to not eat, but must understand that the choice offered is the only choice available for that family meal. It should be made clear the family eats the same thing as a cooperating unit.*

88

-   They can choose to continue arguing and fussing, but must understand that gives the parent the right to ask them to act out in their room, until they feel more comfortable being a cooperative part of the family.

*Teaching children to follow standards of behavior helps them to deal with life as an adult.   Teaching about healthy choices is as much a part of home education as other principles.   Parents naturally teach safety in the streets to protect their children.   Parents may then turn around and buy food that can "hurt" the child physically, because of the general lack of knowledge on the prevention of disease.   Not knowing the "laws" of wellness is one problem this country faces.   However, I frequently hear how parents give in to children and teens who refuse to eat known healthier foods, because it is easier than teaching what is healthy.   Children may have the right to refuse, but parents also have the right to provide **only** healthy food for them to eat if they are hungry.   **The parents of today need to get back the responsibility of parenting!   The parents of today need to look at what they are doing, buying, and teaching, if their children are struggling with mental and physical health!***

Do not be afraid to try new vegetables. People tend to buy the same vegetables week after week. This book is not intended to be a cookbook, but you will find some exciting healthy variations you may not have considered. There are many good health cookbooks available in health food stores, and you should purchase several. *These two suggestions are DELICIOUS and may introduce you to several new vegetables*:

Once the woody peel is cut off jicama, you have a delicious vegetable, cooked or raw as finger food. Shoestring jicama looks and tastes like potatoes. Peel and thinly slice one jicama into strips. In 1 tablespoon sesame oil sauté jicama, 2 cloves crushed garlic, 3 tablespoons chopped red bell pepper, 1/8 teaspoon paprika, and 1/8

89

teaspoon sea salt for 10 minutes (stir frequently). Lightly top with fresh ground black pepper. This is a delicious and unique substitute for potatoes.

Kohlrabi is another unusual vegetable, delicious cooked in salted water for 15 minutes or more, or eaten raw. It is an odd-looking light green vegetable with leaves growing out of a bulb-like stem. The name means cabbage-turnip in German. It is great raw finger food, cut into slivers and put in a salad, or as part of a platter of vegetables, and a zingy dip.

Sometimes vegetables you did not like, but are good for you, can be fixed in different ways you now enjoy. *Try these recipes using familiar vegetables eaten too infrequently:*

GREEN MAYONNAISE is great for special occasions. Blanch ½ bunch spinach leaves, 8 sprigs parsley, and a few celery leaves in 1 cup water (drink, or save left-over for soup). Put 1/8 cup of the liquid in a blender with the greens, 1 large fresh garlic, and 1 teaspoon dried tarragon leaves (or fresh if you have it). Blend 30 seconds at high speed, and add 1 cup any cold-pressed mayonnaise, 2 tablespoons olive oil, seasalt to taste, fresh ground black pepper optional. Spread over sliced tomatoes on a bed of red leaf lettuce. Top with chopped green onions and raw sunflower seeds for a salad they will rave about.

BEET DRESSING is another beautiful dressing for everyday, or special occasions. Combine 8 slices organic canned beets, 1/4 cup beet liquid, 1 tablespoon cider vinegar, 3 tablespoons chopped Spring onions, 3 tablespoons any cold-pressed mayonnaise, and blend thoroughly in a blender. Top any choice of salad vegetables for a new taste and visual treat.

Desserts do not have to be a bad word. *Consider this healthy version of a pumpkin pie:*

Buy a ready-made whole wheat or wheat-free pie crust. Combine: 1 can organic pumpkin, ¾ cup rice or coconut milk, ¼ cup maple syrup, 3 teaspoons pumpkin pie spice, 1 teaspoon seasalt; add this to 2 medium organic eggs, beaten well. Fill crust and cover edges with foil. Bake at 450 degrees for 15 minutes, then 350 degrees for 50-60 minutes. Pie can be healthy!

5. FRUIT

The best way to eat fruit is in **small amounts**, in season, and raw. Fruit is high in simple carbohydrates. Your health will not improve as quickly as you wish if you switch from junk food sweets to a "fruitaholic or juiceaholic" diet. Candida yeast and parasites thrive on the breakdown process of sugar, either from unhealthy candy bars or healthy apples. Fresh fruit is best eaten no more than once or twice daily. It takes too much fruit to make a glass of juice … your Candida yeast and parasites can have a birthday party from all the simple sugar.

Orange *juice* does not contain the valuable bioflavonoids found in the white membrane, so you do not get the food value of the entire orange. Next time you feel like having a glass of orange juice, eat an orange and drink a glass of water! Tremendous quantities of fiber and nutrients are thrown away when fruit or any vegetable is juiced commercially or in your home. DO NOT HAVE YOUR GARBAGE CAN HEALTHIER THAN YOU ARE! I do not buy seedless grapes, because there is valuable nutrition in those fibrous seeds!

The best fruit choices are not excessively sweet. Tart apples, cherries, strawberries, papaya, grapefruit, lemon, and pineapple are all good selections. Seasonal fruit that is naturally ripened and contains a large stone or pit is easily digested and absorbed by the body. Dates, mangoes, papayas, apricots, peaches, avocados, cherries, plums, prunes, and grapes with seeds are all excellent. Naturally ripened fruit is not always easy to find. If you can buy fruit directly from the grower, in season, you have a better chance of getting full nutritional value.

6. FATS AND OILS

Fats, proteins and carbohydrates are the primary sources of energy for the body, supplying fuel for body heat and physical activity. "Calorie" is a term that signifies the amount of energy that is released as heat when food is metabolized. Fats are high caloric foods and yield about nine calories per gram; protein and carbohydrates yield four calories per gram.

A low-fat diet is important to protect your circulatory and digestive systems, as well as weight control; but a fat free diet will make you sick. It is good to skin your chicken, but not good to eliminate *essential fatty acids.* When you consume fat, it should do you some good. The essential fatty acids that break down to produce chemicals called prostaglandins are preserved by the cold-pressing process. Refrigerate all open bottles, because "unrefined" oils can turn rancid.

The two most important fatty acids in human nutrition are linoleic acid from Omega 6 oils and linolenic acid from Omega 3 oils which the body cannot make. Good sources are Black Currant Seed oil, Hemp oil, Borage oil, Flaxseed oil (or ground Flaxseed) sold in health food stores, and Emu oil. Flaxseed oil needs sulfurated protein to break it down in the system, so for improved absorption take with food like soy or whole wheat (not dairy often recommend). Fish oil is just Omega 3, and Evening Primrose is just Omega 6. Research has shown the best therapeutic value is in receiving both. For best utilization, the recommended choice for diabetics is Borage oil.

DO NOT ELIMINATE ESSENTIAL FATTY ACIDS IN YOUR EFFORT TO REDUCE FATS! ESSENTIAL FATTY ACIDS ARE NEEDED FOR HEALTHY GLANDULAR FUNCTION ... A BIG MISTAKE TO ELIMINATE THEM!

Fatty acids are destroyed easily by heat, light, and oxygen, so a diet high in processed foods will be deficient in essential fatty acids. It is best to consume good fats and oils in the form of whole, unprocessed foods such as raw nuts and seeds, whole grains, and cold-pressed oils; and/or take an essential fatty acid supplement.

Sesame oil is best for frying because it does not break down into carcinogenic free radicals as rapidly as other oils when it is heated. Olive oil is good for the liver; use it in salad dressings, with fish or seafood, and in stir frying as often as possible. Olive oil is about 75% monounsaturated fats. Virgin has the most olive taste; then comes extra fine virgin; then refined, made from olives too acidic, or having an "off" flavor. Pure olive oil is a mixture of refined and virgin oils. "Light" is pure olive oil with less virgin oil for only a hint of olive taste, so it is most popular for general cooking. All olive oil is best for the liver; *the least refined is always best.* Virgin olive oil will harden in the refrigerator. I always transfer olive oil into a wide mouth jar so I can easily take out what I want.

Use organic butter (hormone and antibiotic free) instead of margarine. I do not recommend hydrogenated margarine because it is high in free radicals that can be carcinogenic, and can block the body's production of prostaglandins. Many margarine products contain milk. Foods in their natural form are always healthier than processed foods. Butter is rich in a form of Vitamin A that is 300% more than the Vitamin A in fish liver oil. Natural D in butter is equal to 10 quarts of milk and 100 times as effective as a synthetic form. Vitamin F in butter acts like a partner with Vitamin D. Vitamin E in butter is a whole, natural complex. *HORMONE AND ANTIBIOTIC FREE BUTTER IN MODERATION IS A GOOD FOOD, BUT "BETTER BUTTER" IS LOWER IN SATURATED FAT AND HIGHER IN ESSENTIAL FATTY ACIDS. The following delicious recipe stays soft in the refrigerator:*

> *1 pound organic butter - very soft*
> *1 cup water*
> *1 cup mild flavored cold-pressed oil*
> *Blend in a heavy-duty mixer (not a blender), food processor, or use a hand mixer. Place in a closed container and refrigerate. You can make one half recipe and freeze two sticks of butter for later, if you use butter infrequently.*

If you have a milk allergy, sinus or respiratory mucus problems, you should be able to use butter because the allergic properties are not in the fat, nor is butterfat mucus forming.

Do not save and reheat any type of oil. I do not recommend deep fat frying for any food, but if you love French fries, *try these three recipes:*

- *For EACH unpeeled potato: slice like French fries, coat with 2 teaspoons of sesame tahini, and 1/4 teaspoon seasalt. Place on oiled baking sheet and bake 35-40 minutes at 450 degrees, turning several times.*

- *Cut 2 potatoes into 8 lengthwise wedges; soak in cold water 30 minutes; pat dry. Toss with 1 tablespoon olive oil, 2 teaspoons oregano leaves, 1/4 teaspoon sea salt; lay out single layer on baking pan. Bake 400 degree oven 35 - 40 minutes until potatoes are tender and brown; turn once. Sprinkle with fresh ground black pepper, and 2 tablespoons malt vinegar. Toss to mix.*

- *2 small sweet potatoes, peeled*
  1 Tablespoon olive oil
  1/8 teaspoon cayenne
  1/4 teaspoon seasalt
  Heat oven to 450 degrees. Cut potatoes into 3 inch long matchstick shapes. Place in a bowl and pour the olive oil over potatoes; sprinkle with cayenne and seasalt. Using your hands, toss the potato sticks until completely coated with oil. Spread out in a single layer on a baking sheet. Bake about 25 minutes, turning every 10 minutes or so. The sweet potatoes are done when they are tender and almost caramelized; they will not really crisp up like french fries but will have a chewy sweetness.

7. PROTEIN

It is important that you put protein in perspective, both in quantity and quality in your diet. Your protein does not have to be hard-to-digest red meat. A serving of red meat several times a week, or in a soup base is all you should consider, and indeed more than you need. Eat more hormone and antibiotic-free fowl, rabbit, a moderate numbers of organic eggs, fish and occasional seafood, or vegetable proteins like soy, Brewer's Yeast or Spirulina.

Most of us need to greatly reduce our consumption of meats, but not everyone should be a vegetarian. A person does not have to eat red meat, but some vegetarians get very tired if they do not consume a little chicken, eggs, fish, or seafood. THE DECIDING FACTOR IS HOW DO YOU FEEL ON YOUR CURRENT DIET? *If you are eating animal products, or you are a strict vegetarian, this test might show you that you are consuming a diet that does not meet your body's needs:*

> *Dr. William Donald Kelly devised a test to determine an individual's energy needs and the kinds of protein best suited for their specific body chemistry: Take a 50 milligram niacin tablet on an empty stomach first thing in the morning. If a flush of uncomfortable degree (or maybe even hives) develops, that person can handle the digestion of sensible amounts of animal protein. If the tablet produces just a mild warm feeling, the person can eat occasional meat. If no reaction occurs, the diet would be better vegetarian. This test may change as your health changes.*

HERE ARE SOME FACTS ON PROTEIN CHOICES:

- **Eggs** should be free range and free of hormones and antibiotics. An organic egg is a good food because it can produce life; eaten in MODERATION it is a healthy addition to most diets. Eggs should never be eaten raw due to possible bacterial contamination.

95

- **Fish** contains an Omega 3 fatty acid that is not found in significant amounts in any other food, except in supplements. It keeps the protein in your blood from becoming sticky and forming clots. People living in coastal countries, and Eskimos statistically have fewer heart attacks. You should eat fish several times a week. Ocean fish may be safer than local fish due to chemicals and pollution; farm raised fish may contain hormones and antibiotics, or can be genetically engineered.

You should also know that the reason you do not think you like fish is that you may not be fixing it correctly. Overdone, tough and oily tasting fish, is not delicious. The best fish without a strong fish flavor is Haddock, Sole, Flounder, Scrod (baby cod), Orange Roughy, and Tilapia. Be careful of raw fish as it can contain parasites! You can buy **cooked** fish sushi rolls or vegetarian sushi. *Try some of my favorite cooked fish ideas:*

a. *Freshly broiled salmon cooked until it flakes but still has moisture, and the deep pink color is gone. Chinook salmon is higher in fat than silver salmon. Sauté or bake salmon in a little Better Butter, chopped spring onions, and/or chopped fresh garlic. Bake at 350 degrees for 10-15 minutes only. Canned salmon makes great salads, patties, or loaves.*

b. *Haddock is one of the tastiest of the firm white fish; be careful NOT to overcook. Many people do not like fish because it is dry and overcooked. Fix haddock or any other mild fish the same as you would salmon.*

c. *Clam chowder can be made "milk" free with a non-dairy milk like rice milk, or with a tomato base. Use clam sauce on whole grain spaghetti, or spaghetti squash for a change. Clam sauce is easy to make:*

96

Sauté 2 large chopped garlic cloves and 2 tablespoons chopped onion in 1/8 cup olive oil until soft. Add 1/4 cup whole wheat flour or spelt flour, 2 teaspoons basil, 1 bottle clam juice, 2 rounded tablespoons fresh parsley, and cook until thickened. Add 2 cans minced clams with juice (read labels - find one without sugar), and ¼ teaspoon seasalt; heat only - boiling toughens clams. Top with fresh, chopped spring onions and soy parmesan cheese (if the casein in that product is tolerated).

d. *Bottled clam juice and fish fillets turn vegetable soup into bouillabaisse. Bouillabaisse, or fisherman's soup, is a sure hit at dinner. This fancier version can be easily adjusted to feed more people:*

Sauté 2 inches of chopped leek or several Spring onions, and 2 large garlic cloves in 1 tablespoon olive oil for 5 minutes. Add 1 bottle clam juice, 1 small can whole tomatoes chopped up, 2 cups chicken broth, 1 medium cubed potato, 1 medium cubed carrot, 1 medium celery stalk cut up, 2 sprigs of fresh parsley, 2 bay leaves (remove before eating); seasoned with optional amounts of cayenne pepper, thyme, seasalt, and simmer for 30 minutes. Add ¾ pound of any inexpensive fish fillets, ¼ pound cleaned shrimp, ¼ pound scallops, ½ pound clams in the shell (washed thoroughly). Cook another 10 minutes, and enjoy!!! If too thick add more chicken broth.

e. *Sauté any fish fillet and serve on a whole grain hamburger roll; use your imagination and garnish for a* **fabulous fish burger***.*

f. *If you wish to sauté razor clams, pound the necks with a mallet and cook in a little Better Butter for 30 seconds on a side; they will toughen if overcooked.*

g. *Arrange six lightly sea-salted large sole fillets in a single layer on an oiled baking dish. Top with a mixture of 1/2 cup cold-pressed oil mayonnaise and 3 teaspoons natural mustard. Bake 350 degrees for 10-15 minutes depending on thickness of the sole. Any fish fillet can be used.*

h. *Fried seafood is not recommended. It is high in fat, and restaurant fried food could be in rancid oil. The only fried food I eat is an occasional treat of tiny fried oysters, coated with a little seasalt and whole wheat or spelt flour, browned over medium heat in cold-pressed sesame, super canola, or peanut oil. These oils go rancid slower in higher heat than other oils.*

i. *If you do not like plain sardines, add to tomato soup. Too often the good taste of sardines on whole grains crackers is forgotten.*

j. *Fish fillets can be fixed in a variety of ways to satisfy even the skeptical fish eater. Cut fish fillets into one inch chunks and check for bones. Place in a casserole sprayed with oil, and let your imagination CREATE a sauce:*

- Wine, Worcestershire sauce and lime juice
- Mayonnaise and mustard
- Your favorite BBQ sauce
- Curry, Better Butter, and almonds
- Lemon, Better Butter and herbs like basil, sage, thyme, marjoram, parsley, chives
- Better Butter, fresh parsley, lemon and fresh grated ginger root
- Leftover vegetarian spaghetti sauce
- Pesto sauce (from health food stores contains dairy)
- Your favorite salad dressing
- Soy sauce, wine vinegar and lemon juice
- Fresh grated ginger and soy sauce

- Sauté olive oil, onion, garlic, celery, tomato until tender, then add to fish
- Garlic, lemon juice, Dijon mustard, Better Butter; top with fresh ground pepper
- Horseradish mustard
- Fresh or bottled salsa

BE CREATIVE! *Bake in a preheated 350 degree oven for 10-15 minutes depending on the thickness of the chunks. Do not overcook! Be willing to try every kind of fish and seafood, and be surprised by new taste treats!*

- **Chicken** should be skinned, hormone and antibiotic-free. White meat is lower in fat than dark meat. Think plain! There are many chicken recipes that do not use lots of fat, dairy, or sugar in sauces. *Here are some recipe ideas:*

Ground chicken, turkey, emu, ostrich, deer or buffalo meat makes a tasty burger. Add onions, garlic, poultry seasoning, an egg to bind, coat with whole grain crumbs and broil. If you cannot tolerate wheat, toast spelt or another tolerate bread, and make your own crumbs in a blender, or omit crumbs. You can also buy frozen chicken patties in health food stores that make great sandwiches.

Ground chicken, turkey, emu, ostrich, deer or buffalo meat can be combined with egg, onions, garlic, and seasalt, and made into balls. Cook in tomato sauce, and serve over mashed potatoes or pasta.

Pound chicken breasts flat with a mallet and sauté on low heat in Better Butter, five minutes on each side. Top with any combination under "j."

Add curry to your favorite chicken and rice recipe for a taste change.

Make your own breast meat chicken strips, or buy them. Sauté in olive oil on low heat until tender, about 10 minutes on a side. Salt with seasalt as desired, and dip in horseradish mustard, honey mustard, or dip of your choice. This is a favorite with children and teens.

Lay breast chicken fillets on an oiled baking dish, lightly salted with seasalt. Cover with thawed frozen spinach that has been seasoned to taste with your choice of mustard. Cover with a lid and bake at 350 degrees for 45 minutes to 1 hour based on thickness of chicken.

Skin 4 chicken breasts and low-heat sauté in 1 tablespoon cold-pressed sesame or peanut oil with 1 sliced onion. Add 1 can natural chicken broth available at a health food store; season with 1/2 teaspoon each marjoram, basil thyme, and tarragon, 1-2 teaspoons curry (to taste), and 1 tablespoon parsley. Cook about 45 minutes, or until chicken is done. Thicken with cornstarch or arrowroot; serve sauce over brown rice.

*This is great for special occasions: Skin 1 chicken (or use desired parts), sauté in 1/4 cup cold-pressed olive oil, 1 small chopped onion, 2 large garlic cloves, 1/2 teaspoon sea salt, 1 ROUNDED tablespoon oregano leaves, on **medium-low** heat 45 minutes – 1 hour; turn occasionally. Remove chicken; stir in 1 fresh tomato cut in wedges **per person**, and slices of summer squash, just to coat with juices but not to cook. Serve with vegetables around chicken on a platter ... beautiful and delicious!*

Leftover chicken or turkey tastes great in this stir-fry. Cook any whole grain pasta according to directions and drain. In a skillet sauté in olive oil: onion, garlic, celery, parsley, broccoli or any other desired vegetable in amounts appropriate for the number of servings. Add cut up chicken or turkey and the cooked pasta. Season to taste with sea salt, and top with freshly ground black pepper.

100

- **Rabbit** is lower in fat and cholesterol than any other mammal meat, and higher in protein. You can use it in any chicken recipe. Some people are unwilling to try rabbit because the whole pieces remind us of cute bunnies. Have your butcher grind rabbit and use it in any hamburger recipe like chili, spaghetti sauce, or rabbitburger. *I have yet to look at ground rabbit and see a rabbit!* Add sage and salt to ground rabbit (or any ground meat) for delicious low-fat sausage.

- **Turkey** is sometimes a bother, and leftover frozen turkey is not as good as freshly cooked. Have your butcher cut a small hormone and antibiotic-free turkey in half and freezer wrap; when you want turkey, bake a half and eat for lunch and dinner until it is gone. *Leftovers are always welcomed; freeze if not consumed in 24 hours.*

  Melt 2 tablespoons Better Butter in a skillet and low-heat sauté 1/4 cup or more chopped onion, one chopped garlic clove, and 1-1/2 cups unpeeled diced potato for 15 minutes or until soft. Add 2 cups diced chicken or turkey, 1/2 teaspoon salt, and heat through. Mix in 1 cup or more natural chicken broth and 1 tablespoon minced fresh parsley. Add more chicken broth as needed to keep the hash from being dry.

  Make soup out of the turkey carcass by breaking into pieces and covering with filtered salted water. Boil 1 hour, pick out turkey meat and strain broth. Add turkey meat, carrots, celery, parsley, onions, garlic, cubed potato, washed brown rice optional, and poultry seasoning to broth and simmer for 1 hour. If rice is not added, you can add a pasta choice of shape.

- **Eggs** are capable of producing life, and are a perfect food. Buy hormone and antibiotic-free eggs, from a free ranging flock with a rooster, for best nutritional quality.

101

Cholesterol in eggs is over-rated as a cause of high cholesterol in our blood. moderation is the key word. Prepare eggs hard-cooked, soft-cooked, poached, baked, or low heat stove set. An opportunity to use your creativity in preparing eggs is a low-heat omelet:

Wipe a cast iron skillet with sesame oil. Whip 1 tablespoon water and a dash of salt with 2 eggs. Pour into skillet and bake at 350 degrees until set. Place your favorite filling on half the omelet, fold the other half over, and cut in half to serve two. Some foods good in omelets include soy or rice cheese (you can get casein-free soy or rice cheese); salsa; bean sprouts; raw green spring onions; tomatoes; cooked onion, garlic or green peppers; healthy sausage or turkey bacon cooked, blotted dry and crumbled ... or be creative!

- **Emu** is the prized, dark red meat of a flightless bird that tastes like beef, but has the recommendation of the American Heart Association. Emu is available in steaks, but also ground meat. Ostrich is another bird that is available in both ground meat, strips, and steaks, and sold in some health food stores. *These fowl choices can be used any way beef is used, and makes a delicious meatloaf:*

1 pound of Emu or Ostrich meat, 1 egg, 1/2 cup soy or rice milk (this keeps it from being too firm), optional 1 slice toasted tolerated bread put into the blender to make crumbs, 2 sprigs of chopped fresh parsley, chopped onion based on personal taste, 2 large chopped garlic, season with seasalt to taste, and top with a thick layer of organic ketchup. Place in oiled baking dish, cover and bake 350 degrees for 1 hour.

- **Duck** is a wonderful change for holiday meals. Because of very thick skin, duck is high in fat, and too greasy to enjoy unless you skin the duck. *For an unforgettable special event dinner:*

Place skinned duck in roaster pan. Surround with quartered unpeeled organic potatoes. Mix together 1 can organic orange juice concentrate, 1 can water, 1 teaspoon dry mustard, 2 tablespoons honey, 1 tablespoon Worcestershire sauce, ¼ teaspoon seasalt. Adjust seasonings in sauce to taste. Add to duck and potatoes; bake covered at 350° for 2 ½ hours. Baste hourly, turning duck. Fabulous!

- **Buffalo or deer meat** is a good substitute for the more allergenic beef. Both are firm, less fatty meat than beef. Both can be used for meatloaf, hamburgers, tacos, or any other use of hamburger. Buffalo and deer meat are both available farm raised, and sold in some health food stores. *They are both hard to digest red meat, so eat in moderation only if you are hydrated, and your pH is within normal range.*

8. DAIRY PRODUCTS

Healthiest milk is non-fat; preferably non-fat soured forms such as yogurt, kefir, and buttermilk. However, since milk is an extremely allergenic food and mucus forming, I suggest you eliminate all milk and dairy products from your diet for four days. Then do a test meal as outlined in this chapter. Friendly bugs in dairy yogurt help with digestion, form colonies that manufacture some B vitamins, and push out unwanted bacteria and Candida yeast. Soy yogurt available in health food stores has the same good bacteria, without the problems associated with dairy products.

If you reduce meat, soft drinks and processed foods in your diet, your body's calcium need would most likely be satisfied by non-dairy sources of calcium like seeds and nuts, dark green vegetables, fish and seafood, seaweeds, beans, egg yoke, chicken, molasses, carob flour, or soy products. *You might try adding a little maple syrup and pecans to plain vanilla soy yogurt.* **Keep dairy products for social occasions only.**

9. NUTS AND SEEDS

"Seeds contain nearly every single food element that has been discovered. and doubtless all the additional factors not yet identified. No other one food is so rich in nutrients as the seed, containing as it does the life forces needed to build the new generation. Seeds have highly potent therapeutic values."

- Dr. Bernard Jensen

Tucked inside every seed is the secret of life. Seeds provide the body with vitamins, minerals, proteins, trace elements, and the right kind of essential fatty acids. Look for every opportunity to use seeds in soups, casseroles, sauces, breads, muffins, waffles, pancakes, salads, salad dressings, blender drinks, and sprinkled on almost anything you can imagine. You may eat a few small fruit seeds from apples and grapes; larger quantities like cantaloupe and watermelon can be blended in any liquid and strained to make a delicious drink. Dr. Jensen warns that apple seeds from heavily sprayed orchards can contain up to 75 percent of the spray. Organically grown food is always best.

Nuts and seeds should be eaten fresh and raw, except peanuts, which are legumes and must NOT be eaten raw. Commercial oil-roasted nuts and seeds are often prepared in rancid oil at high temperatures, so dry roasted is better; raw is best.

Nuts and seeds should be stored in the freezer, as they turn rancid quickly. Nuts in the shell should be consumed quickly, or frozen. Nuts will not freeze solid due to the high fat content, and can be eaten right from the freezer. *Do not buy broken nuts or products with broken nuts, as they can become rancid before the package is even opened.* Rancid oils are hard on the liver; never eat any nut or seed that tastes rancid.

Nuts contain large amounts of high quality protein and beneficial essential fatty acids. They are high in fat, so they should be consumed in small amounts. Eight to ten nuts (or what you can fit in the palm of your hand) at a time are recommended for good digestion. Remember..."*Too much of a good thing does not make it better!*" You can have more nuts after a few hours. Hazelnuts, macadamia nuts, pecans, almonds and pistachios are high in monounsaturated fats. I do not recommend nut butter if you have a severe reaction to any nut or peanut. Equipment cross used for different butters may contain trace amounts of unlisted nuts or peanuts.

Some people prefer the nut butters, and these should be used up quickly when opened. *A favorite lunch or snack is:*

Put a brown rice cake in the oven at 200 degrees for ten minutes to crisp. Wrap in foil if you are taking it to work. When ready, top with a layer of almond butter or any nut butter available in health food stores, or fresh ground peanut butter available now in some grocery stores ... Top that with banana slices if desired ... DELICIOUS!

Nut or seed milk is a SUPERIOR calcium substitute for milk, and can be used in any recipe for added nutrition. This lacks milk sugar so recipes like muffins, pancakes or waffles need added natural sugar like pure maple syrup to brown. *To make nut or seed milk ...*

*Mix 2 teaspoons of Tahini (ground sesame seeds), **OR** ¼ cup almonds (or other bland tasting nut) in 1 cup water in a blender. Blend until a fine liquid.*

Sprouting seeds improves their nutritive value. Sprouts are the most ALIVE food we can put into our bodies, and you do not need a farm to sprout seeds! All you need to become an organic gardener is enthusiasm, and room to set a small pan in the light.

Get one of the many fine books available on seed sprouting techniques. You can sprout grass seed purchased from pet shops, and give your indoor cats the grass he or she loves. HAPPY SPROUTING ... THE REWARDS ARE TERRIFIC!

10. WATER

Water is the #1 health problem in the world! The true meaning of a preventive approach to health care is to first exclude the simpler causes of disease, and then think of the more complicated. The simple truth is that dehydration can cause any symptom or disease.

Dehydration eventually causes loss of function; various "signals" called symptoms have been considered the indicators of disease. Instead of providing water for these "signals," modern medicine silences them with drugs. **REMEMBER TO FIRST DO NO HARM. CONSUME EIGHT GLASSES OF PURE, FILTERED WATER DAILY** (or one ounce of filtered water for each two pounds of body weight).

City water, even well water in our chemical society contains chemicals the liver must detoxify. Water from *ANY SOURCE* should be put through some purification system. Since you absorb 60 percent of what goes on your skin, a shower or bath can put unwanted chemicals into the body. Showering with chlorine can cause dull, brittle hair; flaky scalp; burning eyes; dry skin; skin rashes; and hot chlorine-filled steam invading your lungs. When chlorine combines with organic matter in water, volatile pollutants like chloroform are formed, which can cause liver and kidney damage, depression, and is a suspected carcinogen.

Reverse osmosis is a recommended form of filtering water, because it back washes the filter. Distilled water is also recommended over filters that do not completely filter out all the unwanted elements. Your healthy diet and/or supplements can replace loss minerals in both reverse osmosis and distilled water. Inexpensive filters that do not remove amoeba parasites are not recommended. Most filtered water is "dead water," and new technology is returning energy to filtered water.

Highly recommended book: *YOUR BODY'S MANY CRIES FOR WATER* by F. Batmangheilidj, M.D.

[] [] [] [] []

SOME FOOD FACTS AND
SUBSTITUTIONS IN COOKING

This section is not intended to be complete in the area of food allergies and substitutions. It is meant to make you more aware of the possible cause of your symptoms being a food allergic reaction. *I have listed only a few examples, but it could get you thinking in the right direction.*

CORN ALLERGY:

Sensitivity to corn is one of the most common food allergies, and the most difficult food in the diet to avoid. Allergic symptoms can be as the result of ingestion, inhalation or contact. Corn is used in a great variety of foods, and may not always be listed on the label. Corn can be as hidden as the glue on the back of stamps. If you crave corn in any form and eat it on a regular basis, suspect an allergy. Start reading labels for corn free products, and observe what you are exposed to if you have symptoms. Being a good detective can pay off matching symptoms with exposures.

Arrowroot is a substitute for corn in thickening.

WHEAT ALLERGY:

Wheat contains two allergic fractions ... gluten and starch. Gluten may cause the most problems focusing on the stomach or intestines. However, a gluten reaction can affect other parts of the body, like painful ribs after eating gluten.

For gluten sensitivity avoid the following:

> Wheat flour or durum wheat
> Graham flour, gluten flour, enriched flour
> Hydrolyzed vegetable protein, monosodium glutamate
> Barley, oats, rye
> Triticale, Amaranth
> Buckwheat (a non-grain with a gluten like protein, that may be tolerated by some gluten sensitive people)
> Spelt

Non-gluten substitutes:

> Potato and sweet potato
> Soy, tofu
> Rice and all gluten free rice products
> Corn and all gluten free corn products
> Millet, Quinoa
> Tapioca, arrowroot
> All legumes
> Spaghetti squash

Substitutes for wheat used as a binder in recipes are egg, gluten free rice bread, agar agar (a seaweed gelatin), tapioca, or mashed potatoes.

MILK ALLERGY:

Milk has a highly allergic potential that is too often missed by our dairy and beef oriented society. It should be considered a possible cause of your symptoms if any form of it is a serious staple in your diet. You can keep an allergy going if you have it once in four days, so just reducing dairy or beef is not going to eliminate allergic stress. Dairy and beef are often hidden in supplements, in beef capsules, and skin care products.

In ingredients, avoid all milk in any form, all milk products in any form, most margarine, whey, casein (including Goat's milk), lactalbumin, beef, veal, gelatin and glycerin (unless

108

vegetarian). Butter is alright because it does not contain protein, and is not mucus forming. Substitutes for capsules are vegicaps or softgels. Substitutes for milk include soy, rice, coconut, and almond milk.

SOY ALLERGY:

This allergy is difficult because it is in many health products and is often a substitute for dairy. You need to read labels very carefully, or even call the company if you want to take a certain supplement. When it comes to soy, dairy, or corn allergies, keep your food list to simple products you know are safe.

Rice milk is not high enough in fat to be a substitute for soy in babies under three years old. Rice or soy cheese with casein is not dairy free. Look for casein free cheeses.

BLACK PEPPER:

This is a frequent unrecognized allergen. I know one person who had suicidal attempts traced to black pepper, and another person who fell into a deep sleep after eating black pepper. Again, if you crave a food, use it regularly, and are unhappy if you do not have it, you should suspect an allergy causing one of your symptoms.

Consider seasoning power with chili powder, or cayenne pepper.

PEANUTS:

This may seem an obvious food to eliminate, but many restaurants cook with peanut oil. Peanut is a legume, and should never be eaten raw. Peanut is in the same family with soy.

[] [] [] [] []

BREAKFAST OR BRUNCH SUGGESTIONS

The body works in rhythms that allow certain functions to perform best during certain times. *It is called Circadian Rhythm and if you acknowledge the cycles, it could have a positive effect on your health:*

Nutrient Ingestion - Digestion. . . . . .noon to 8PM
Nutrient Distribution - Utilization - Rest. . . .8PM to 4AM
Waste Elimination. 4AM to noon

With all the elements of health stacked against our modern society, it could be beneficial for you to eat light before noon. What you eat is important in the digestive process. Hard-to-digest, high-fat red meat like sausage is not recommended before noon. Small amounts of easy-to-digest foods, especially high fiber foods like whole grains that jump-start your intestines, liquids, and fresh fruit that gives you energy, are all good choices first thing in the morning. At least choose to have your eggs or lean meat sausage for a late breakfast (brunch).

Some suggestions listed may not be perfect food combining, or even considered healthy choices by a pure health enthusiast. However, this book is for people wanting to *start* making healthy changes without alienating the family, or shocking themselves. For some people, it is like the first few baby steps ... learning to get better one step at a time. *If you drink a glass of filtered water 1/2 hour before you eat, work on pH balance and other digestion principles discussed in the Digestion chapter, relax during mealtime and chew your food well, you will digest "healthy" food better.* Some people who are very ill may need to follow *stricter food combining rules;* some people are more motivated than others to follow perfect recommendations. *For the majority reading this book, these suggestions will be a helpful beginning to start making better choices. Remember, the harder to digest choices should be eaten as a late breakfast, or brunch selection:*

1. Whole wheat waffles or pancakes can be made in double batches and leftovers frozen. Warm, and top with maple syrup, Better Butter; optional chopped nuts or seeds.

2. Cut toasted whole wheat bread into cubes and mix with an organic soft-cooked egg and sea salt.

3. Rushed mornings may require on-the-road selections. Consider an organic hard-boiled egg, a piece of fresh fruit, a few nuts, or a muffin. You can top a whole grain muffin with Better Butter, freshly ground peanut butter, nut butters, fruit juice sweetened organic fruit jams, organic apple or pumpkin butters.

4. Stretch your imagination and "create" a vegetable omelet.

5. Cut up an orange or a grapefruit and top with a little maple syrup and sunflower seeds; or add water to make a blender drink. Seeds get bitter if they are ground too long.

6. Scrambled eggs will be lighter if you beat in 1 tablespoon soy or rice milk for each egg; pinch of sea salt. Melt 1 teaspoon Better Butter for each egg in pan, and cook eggs on low heat. Serve with whole grain toast.

7. Make your favorite whole grain muffin recipe on your day off, and freeze. Set several muffins out to thaw before you go to bed; 30 seconds in the microwave, or warm in the oven or toaster the next morning gets you going. Add a piece of fresh fruit. *Instead of muffins make this excellent zucchini bread:*

   Cream 1/2 cup butter and 1/2 cup honey. Beat in 2 large eggs. Add 1 cup grated, packed raw zucchini and 1 teaspoon natural vanilla extract. Add 2 cups whole wheat flour, 2 1/2 teaspoons baking powder, 1 teaspoon ground cinnamon, full 1/2 teaspoon sea salt. Beat well until mixed. Bake in 8 inch square sprayed pan at 350 degree oven for 30-40 minutes.

8. Leftover mashed or sliced baked potato, or brown rice can be low-heat sautéed in a small amount of Better Butter, with or without an egg, and topped with a few seeds or chopped nuts.

   Leftover food should preferably be eaten in 24 hours, and can be "revived" with fresh parsley, spring onions, and garlic.

9. If your high-energy morning work requires a "hearty" breakfast, you can make your own low-fat sausage with ground hormone and antibiotic-free fowl meat, or rabbit, add sage to taste, and solar sea salt. Add fresh ground black pepper *at the table* if you wish, but cooked pepper is hard on the liver. Ground pepper can turn rancid, so always grind whole peppercorns as needed.

10. Tapioca does not need to be a milk base; for one serving of fruit tapioca soak 1/8 cup Minute Tapioca in 1/2 cup fresh orange juice, 2 teaspoons pure maple syrup (or more based on sweetness of orange), 1/2 cup water, and a dash of salt for 5 minutes. Bring to a boil and simmer 5 minutes; let stand 10 minutes. Eat warm, topped with a few chopped pecans; great for a relaxing weekend morning change.

11. Chill and slice cooked cereal. *Buy Polenta from the health food store, or make as follows: .*

    Mix 1 cup cornmeal with 1/2 cup cold water. Heat 2 cups water with 1/2 teaspoon salt in a double boiler. Stir in cornmeal and cook until thickened, stirring occasionally. Cook covered on very low heat for 20-30 minutes. Pour into a loaf pan and chill. Slice and warm in a little Better Butter, serve topped with a small amount of maple syrup, and chopped nuts or seeds.

12. Oatmeal, whole wheat, brown rice, rye or buckwheat cooked cereal, topped with pure maple syrup, finely chopped almonds or pecans, and rice or soy milk. Health food stores carry some nutritious, chemical free dry cereal that is delicious with maple syrup and mild tasting vanilla rice milk, or stronger soy milk.

[] [] [] [] [] []

EXCITING LUNCH SUGGESTIONS NEXT

1. Whole wheat or corn tortillas with heated vegetarian chili (canned or homemade), sprouts, and shredded soy or rice cheese (if casein tolerated) may be rolled up burrito-style, or heat in a Quesadilla maker.

2. Small baked white or sweet potatoes are delicious topped with a little Better Butter and a few nuts or seeds. Add Better Butter and cinnamon to sweet potatoes for a real taste treat!

3. Make enough soup to freeze 3-4 quarts; thaw for lunches, or dinner. I have a "soup making" day as needed and make several recipes that day. It is a real project, but the rewards are great with a freezer stocked for months. *I make most soup recipes in the oven so the soup does not burn:*

    BUTTER BEAN SOUP: put 1 package navy beans soaked per routine, in 2 quarts filtered water, 2 LARGE chopped onions, 4 LARGE carrots, and 3 teaspoons seasalt in a large oven proof container. Bake at 325 degrees for 3 hours or until tender; add 4 tablespoons Better Butter.

113

PEA SOUP: Soak 1 package split peas over night and drain. Cook until soft in 2 quarts filtered water, 1 medium diced onion, 1 large stalk celery, 2 bay leaves (remove before blending at the end of cooking), 2 large garlic cloves, 3 diced carrots, ½ tsp. thyme, ½ tsp. rosemary, ½ tsp. oregano, and 1 large cubed potato. Add 1 pound of turkey bacon cooked, blotted dry, and crumbled to soup. When peas are soft, place by the cupful into a blender and whirl just enough to make into a smooth but still slightly textured soup.

4. Leftover turkey or chicken make great salads or sandwiches.

5. Unsalted, natural corn chips can be topped with fresh salsa, chopped green onions, and soy or rice cheese (if casein tolerated) melted on top for healthy *nachos*. Remember to try the casein-free cheeses in health food stores, available in both cheddar and mozzarella.

6. Sardines in water mixed with mayonnaise and onion mustard on whole grain crackers.

7. Vegetarian eggrolls, whole wheat chicken pies, natural chicken or turkey hot dogs and lunch meats are available at health food stores. Large size hot dog brands are juicier than those brands with eight in a package.

8. An all natural hot dog, some sprouts, and fresh salsa on a whole wheat or spelt roll is a substantial lunch. Make healthier hot dog sauce with any combination of natural ketchup, cold-pressed mayonnaise, natural mustard, and naturally sweetened pickle relish. If you cannot eat wheat, spread sauce on a corn tortilla, large romaine lettuce or Chinese cabbage leaf, and fold around your hot dog. Also, add hot dogs to tomato soup.

9. Soy or rice cheese may be melted on a whole wheat or corn tortilla, topped with chopped scallions, tomatoes, sprouts, green peppers, and sunflower seeds and served immediately. Substitute vegetarian chili for the cheese if you cannot tolerate any form of cheese.

10. A squash cut in half (butternut is consistently sweet and delicious), and baked for one hour or more at 350 degrees, topped with Better Butter, sunflower seeds, and sea salt is a great addition to any meal. For a variation, scoop cooked squash into a saucepan, add Better Butter, sea salt, and cinnamon for a surprising taste treat.

11. Cook a few baked potatoes, sweet potatoes, and a butternut squash cut in half, all at the same time. Put into individual refrigerator containers, and when you want a hot, quick snack, heat your choice, and season as desired. You could sauté an egg, or eat fish or chicken with either the white or sweet potato. *This sweet potato biscuit recipe is delicious, and easy to make with your stored cooked sweet potatoes:*

    Blend 1 cup whole wheat flour, 1/4 cup dark brown sugar, 1 tablespoon baking powder, and 3/4 teaspoon sea salt. Cut in 1/4 cup butter until mixture is consistency of corn meal. Add 1 cup mashed cooked sweet potato, and 1/8 cup rice or soy milk; mix to form a soft dough. Turn out on a lightly floured board, and knead gently for 10 seconds. Roll to 1/2 inch thickness; cut biscuits with a 2 inch biscuit cutter, or use the top of a glass. Bake about 14 minutes on a oil coated cookie sheet, 450 degrees.

12. Chopped scallions and an egg added to shredded zucchini, lightly salted, and coated with whole wheat or spelt flour makes a tasty pancake. Sprinkle with paprika and sauté at medium heat in a little sesame or peanut oil.

You can make extra of these at dinner, and heat at lunch. Top with organic unsweetened applesauce.

13. A good tofu cookbook is a helpful addition to your home library. One of my favorites is a tofu Reuben sandwich:

   Spread two slices of whole grain rye bread (or any tolerated bread) generously with your favorite salad dressing. Sauté 2 slices of tofu 1/2 inch thick in Better Butter, and place on bread. Top with soy or rice cheese; broil until melted. Top with heated sauerkraut and dashes of soy sauce. Top with the second piece of bread and ENJOY ... DELICIOUS! Do not count this out if you cannot tolerate the casein in the cheese. This recipe is delicious with casein free rice cheese.

14. Add 1 tablespoon Better Butter and 1/4 cup water to a medium peeled, 1/2 inch sliced eggplant, a medium chopped onion, and 2 chopped garlic cloves in a skillet. Lightly sprinkle with sea salt, and steam 15 minutes on each side, or until soft; add any non-dairy pasta sauce. Serve topped with raw sunflower seeds. This is *great* for lunch or a light dinner.

15. Warm wheat or corn tortillas in a skillet or Quesadilla maker, and top with warmed hormone and antibiotic free chicken or turkey bologna. Top that with any cold-pressed mayonnaise, relish from the health food store, and honey mustard. Roll up and enjoy!!!

16. Any meatloaf left over from dinner makes a great sandwich.

17. The best lunch is to start drinking your blender drink, so read on!

[] [] [] [] [] []

HEALTHY BLENDER DRINK

One example of SUPER FOOD is a blender drink that contains the best vitamins, minerals, protein, and supplements to give you energy, and keep you nourished for hours. The amount can be anywhere from one cup to one quart. It is a perfect choice for people who eat too fast and have poor digestion, for people who have to eat out a lot, for people who are too busy sometimes to stop for lunch, or for people tired of planning their lunch. Some combinations may not have taste appeal for you, and others are delicious. Be willing to experiment to find your favorites. *The following guidelines will help you with selection options:*

BASE LIQUID includes any combination of the following:

- 1 up to 3 cups of filtered water.

- ½ cup of soy, rice, or almond milk ... or

- ½ up to 1 cup of any health food store brand of vegetable juice (preferably organic) ... or

- ½ cup organic fruit juice, 1 tablespoon fruit concentrate, or one piece of fresh fruit. Fruit should be considered your fruit for the day, and is the best choice for a breakfast blender drink. A small amount of fruit, or organic juice can be added to blender drinks with vegetables to improve the taste. *A vegetable drink will always taste better if you add ½ fresh lemon or lime, or 1 tablespoons pure lemon or lime juice with no preservatives.* A palatable blender drink full of alive enzymes *consumed,* is better than perfect food combining drink that is *not consumed. Protein in blender drinks is easier to digest, and not the same problem of combining fruit with harder to digest proteins.*

117

SUPPLEMENT OPTIONS ADDED TO BLENDER DRINKS:

- a scoop of any non-dairy protein powder.

- greens or algae powder like spirulina, blue-green algae, wheat or barley grass.

- 1 scoop Glutamine powder that nutritionally supports your immune function, and intestinal health. Glutamine is the most prevalent amino acid in the body, assisting in absorption of other amino acids.

- A blender drink is a good way to get essential fatty acid oils. You can include 1 tablespoon pressure sealed ground Flaxseed (always refrigerated after opening pressure sealed pouch). Ground Flaxseed is better than Flaxseed oil because it also contains the fiber. Flaxseed is best absorbed if taken with protein.

OPTIONAL ADDITIONS: Buffered Vitamin C powder, apple pectin powder (circulatory cleanser), liquid herbal iron (from health food stores, if you have nail ridges), one teaspoon sesame tahini or almond butter (for added calcium), or one tablespoon lecithin granules (to aid fat digestion). Only add supplements that make the drink taste pleasant. This IS a meal substitute and should be enjoyed.

VEGETABLES IN LUNCH OR DINNER BLENDER DRINK:

Add small amounts of five-six raw vegetables (organic if available) to blender. Examples: *small piece raw beet (or powdered beet crystals available in some health food stores), several sprigs of fresh parsley, leaf of lettuce (darker foods contain more nutrients; romaine lettuce has twice the calcium and iron, eight times Vitamin C, and 10+ times Vitamin A as iceberg lettuce), leaf of chinese cabbage, one-two radishes, one half or one carrot depending on size, one half stalk celery, leaf of kale or other greens, several slices of summer squash or cucumber, slice of turnip, or any other vegetable EXCEPT onions or garlic because of the strong mouth odor they leave. Potatoes, beans, and peas are not good blender choices partly because they thicken the drink.*

I do not add fresh tomatoes to any fruit base, because it gives me a *taste* change from the tomato vegetable base drink. Too many vegetables will make the drink thick; the amount should equal a *large* salad. Vegetables that should be steamed before blending include asparagus, cauliflower, cabbage, spinach and broccoli. Most vegetables can be added raw. If you are in doubt, ask the produce manager, or a manager in a health food store.

If you have never eaten a certain vegetable, do not know how to prepare it, or do not like (or think you do not like) the taste of a certain vegetable, the blender drink is a perfect way to consume foods without any single taste dominating. *You do not have to know how to prepare any vegetable; only that you wash it, store in a glass jar, large plastic container, or zip-lock bag, and put a small amount in the blender drink.* WOW, HOW SIMPLE!!! Once you get the routine established, it will take you about five minutes to make a healthy, nutritious blender drink that you can use for a meal replacement, or a quart drink to consume throughout the day. You can carry your blender drink in a car cooler, and enjoy a nutrition break anytime.

ROTATE ALL SELECTIONS! Do **not** buy the same vegetables you bought the last trip to the grocery store. Eating a wide variety of vegetables is easy with the blender drinks. *Rotation of vegetables, and all other food, is beneficial for these reasons:*

- **Prevention of allergies or intolerance to chemicals in food.** *You are less likely to develop allergies to foods you do not eat everyday. Some foods may be staples to you, but you are missing a lot of healthy foods when you become dependent on just a few.*

- **Balancing your nutrients.** *Foods vary in proportions of nutrients; if you tend to eat the same things daily, you* *may be eating too much of some nutrients, and not enough of others. A limited selection will most likely produce imbalances and deficiencies. BALANCE is an important word to remember.*

- **More interesting diet.** *Not everyone will make blender drinks with all the unusual vegetables nicely rotated. Some people eat lettuce, tomato and cucumber salads, and when they run out of those vegetables they purchase more lettuce, tomatoes and cucumbers. Getting stuck in too many dietary routines could represent the same pattern in your daily life, and prevent you from enjoying challenges. You can learn to eat most any reasonable food. All dietary habits started out with you making choices. New choices can be as comfortable as old choices in time.*

VARIATION TO QUART
VEGETABLE BLENDER DRINK:

To eight ounces of any flavor soy, rice or almond milk plus eight ounces of water, add any choice of the following: one tablespoons Lewis Laboratory Brewer's Yeast, one tablespoon any nut butter or peanut butter, two teaspoons beet crystals (optional), one tablespoon ground Flaxseed, one scoop of non-dairy protein powder, one scoop Glutamine powder, or any other nutritional liquid or powder supplement you are taking at the time. Carry with you in a *hard* plastic container, and drink ½ at a time for a quick energy boost, or meal replacement. Plastic containers for carrying liquids should be hard plastic and not able to be squeezed, so the phenol does not gas out of the plastic into your drink. You can get hard plastic containers in stores that carry camping equipment. Some health food stores sell hard plastic containers for water purchase. This is important because the liver cannot detoxify phenol. Do not pay money for filtered water you think is healthy, but is chemically contaminated with phenol.

EXTRA FOOD TO EAT WITH YOUR BLENDER DRINK:

Nuts and seeds, whole grain breads and crackers, soy dairyless yogurt, rice or soy cheese if casein tolerated (or casein free products), one piece fresh fruit, or any healthy snack choice if you are still hungry.

EQUIPMENT TO MAKE BLENDER DRINKS

EQUIPMENT:

The best choice is a HEAVY DUTY blender like Osterizer Classic, with stainless steel sides and a high/low switch. Do not buy a blender with multiple speeds because it is harder to keep clean. The Vita-Mix is more expensive (800-VITAMIX) but helpful if you make bread. Blender drinks are better than *juicing* vegetables because of the retained fiber, and the ability to add other ingredients.

I love my blender drinks on the five working days, sitting on my desk next to a glass of filtered water. The drink allows me to keep a steady pace without ups and downs, and still feel good at the end of the day. People who travel by car can take their quart blender drink, and extra food options in a cooler, any day or every day. It sure beats a fast food stop for meals ... and questionable nutrition. On the weekend I have other options that provides a change of pace, so the routine does not get boring.

HELP FOR SHOPPING

1. Read labels on everything you buy and look for hidden sources of sugars, refined flour, and chemical additives.

2. Check your cupboard for canned goods, and evaluate whether these products could be purchased fresh, lower sodium levels, less chemical additives, lower fat, and lower

sugar. Some products like tuna or sardines can be purchased in the grocery store, but products like vegetarian chili, tomato sauce, chicken broth, soup, and beans may be best purchased from a health food store. Grocery stores are starting natural food sections, so more things will be available there. Ask your store manager to stock what you want. *Grocery stores will carry what is often requested.*

3. Purchase a recipe file box for your favorite healthy food recipes. Favorite family recipes that do not contain the best health ingredients, or the best food combining choices, are okay for special occasions. Keep only those special favorites, and discard the rest.

4. Eliminate purchases of new foods containing:

Artificial color	Refined flour	Sodium Nitrate
Artificial flavoring	Monosodium glutamate	BHA
Refined sugar	Sodium Nitrite	BHT

5. Purchase a pressure cooker, and a Quesadilla maker for quick nutritious meals.

6. Collect large glass jars to store washed vegetables in refrigerator. When you purchase zip-lock bags get the kind that has the "zipper," and not just matching the strips. Purchase large plastic sealed containers for storage.

7. Purchase a heavy-duty blender if you do not have one. It is an investment in your future.

8. Replace aluminum cookware with stainless steel, Corning Ware, or iron. Buy aluminum-free baking powder.

9. Get a filter for your well or city drinking water, and a shower filter for city water. Keep current on ways new technology improves water energy and filtration.

10. Purchase a stainless steel eight quart pasta cooker/steamer. This size is big enough to make soup.

11. Purchase cookbooks geared to more healthy eating; especially reducing sugar, fat, red meat, dairy products, and refined grains.

12. Put a "To Buy" shopping note paper on your refrigerator door so you can jot down special needs as you remember.

13. Purchase an assortment of nuts and seeds to eat as snacks or use in meal planning, and store in the freezer.

14. Purchase cold-pressed oils high in monounsaturated fat like olive, flaxseed, almond, avocado, or peanut. Keep refrigerated after opening.

15. Purchase natural sugars like honey, maple syrup, and molasses. Also have on hand a small supply of better sugars for those special needs, like sucanat, fructose, or the non-caloric stevia.

16. Purchase whole wheat or spelt flour, brown rice, organic oats, and other grains; keep all grains in the refrigerator. There is some protein loss freezing bread, but whole grain breads will mold if stored even in the refrigerator for a long period.

17. Purchase a healthier version of stock food supplies from the health food store such as catsup, mayonnaise, mustard, relish, salsa, chicken stock, tomato soup, and sea salt, to mention only a few. This turnover may need to be gradual because of finances, but you do have purchasing power on new items.

[] [] [] [] []

So, you want to feel good, and enjoy life ...

Good nutrition is the best place to start. The first stage of deficiency begins when you mishandle food, make poor selections, fail to digest your food, or fail to utilize your digested food. You live or die on a cellular basis; when the supply of nutrients stops, your needs are drawn from your reserves. If the nutrients are not available, your body shows signs of stress with symptoms like indigestion, irritability and depression. If you had a pain in your side today, but did not have it yesterday, and the doctor said you had colon cancer, you did not know yesterday you had a serious illness. You were developing colon cancer for five to twenty years, and did not know it. *To have no symptoms is not an indication of health.* Any symptom is your body telling you that you have not been as well as you thought, and you are now in a state of crisis. If you are treated symptomatically, as I was, you keep getting sicker.

I have just touched the surface with the information available on the subject of nutrition. This is a LIFETIME study, and the more books and newsletters you obtain, the more knowledgeable you will become.

Do not feel pressured in your "wellness life journey." You will continually learn new things that will add to your overall knowledge. My 23 years of learning have been a constant source of pleasure ... and I am still learning.

When you rely on social pressures, advertisements, and family habits to "inform" you on facts that affect your well being, you may be unhappy with the direction of your health. Assuming responsibility for your health means YOU become aware of what it takes to allow the body to work at optimum performance or heal itself. *After you make these beginning changes, you can become more strict, if that is your choice.*

We love to blame our poor health on heredity, but the influence of heredity is minimal compared to nutrition. The basic condition that makes our cells vulnerable to disease is inadequate nutrition. When the nutritional balance of the body is restored through hydration, proper digestion, absorption and

124

metabolism of healthy food, the "power to heal" begins your health metamorphosis.

Diet is what you put into your mouth; nutrition is what your cells actually receive. That means good digestion so you get the most from the food you eat... so dear reader ... read on ...

CHAPTER 3

DIGESTION

YOU EAT TO LIVE ... NOT LIVE TO EAT. YOU LIVE OR DIE ON A CELLULAR BASIS, AND WHAT YOU EAT DETERMINES CELLULAR HEALTH. YOU DERIVE NO VALUE FROM FOODS THAT ARE NOT DIGESTED.

Of the three major life-sustaining nutrients ... protein, carbohydrates, and fat ... the chemical structures of protein are the most fundamental. Proteins alone serve as the building blocks out of which all the cells of our bodies are constructed; the other two factors are used principally as energy sources. Without protein, the human body would not exist.

Proteins, carbohydrates, and fats ingested as meat, bread, fruit, or other food are not usable by the body in that form. Changes that happen to food as it is affected by different enzymes, refine the food into nutrients that can be used by the cells.

This process of disintegrating and refining of food is called DIGESTION. It is partly mechanical as in chewing, swallowing, and churning of foods. It is also partly the changes foods undergo as they are affected by proteins known as enzymes. The basic process of digestion is the splitting of a compound into fragments by enzymes specific for each type of food; and each enzyme has well-defined limitations.

IT IS POSSIBLE THAT EVERY KNOWN DEGENERATIVE DISEASE MAY HAVE ITS ORIGIN IN ENZYME DEFICIENCY. It is estimated that the human body requires about 600 various enzymes to maintain proper health. *COOKING DESTROYS ALL NATURAL ENZYMES, AND REQUIRES THE BODY TO PROVIDE ALL THE ELEMENTS OF DIGESTION.*

❑ ❑ ❑ ❑ ❑ ❑

A WALK THROUGH THE DIGESTIVE PROCESS

Taking the journey with our food, from the time it enters the mouth to the last stage of digestion, is a fascinating story from beginning to end. The digestive process changes carbohydrates to simple sugars called monosaccharides, proteins to amino acids, and fats to fatty acids. It all begins with your first bite of food.

CARBOHYDRATES

Carbohydrates start digesting in the mouth. The three major sources of carbohydrates in the human diet are:

1. *Sucrose - refined sugar*
2. *Lactose - milk sugar*
3. *Starches - complex carbohydrates present in many foods like white potatoes, sweet potatoes, beans, and grains*

Only **starch** digestion begins in the **alkaline** mouth from the **ptyalin** enzyme in the saliva. The combinations of food you eat can affect the quality of this process. An acid food eaten with a starch can change the mouth to *ACIDIC*, and prevent the ptyalin from starting starch digestion in the mouth.

> *You can experience the digestive effect of ptyalin by chewing bread for several minutes. It becomes sweet from the liberation of sugars.*

The action of ptyalin continues in the stomach until the food is completely mixed with gastric juices, which are acidic. Starch digestion stops at this time, and completes the process in the *ALKALINE* small intestine. Before starches enter the liver, they are simple sugars called monosaccharides.

127

PROTEINS

Proteins are fragmented in the digestive tract into complex chains of amino acids. Just like the composition of a word from our alphabet letters, amino acids (the letters) at the cellular level begin to form new proteins (the words), which become new cells in the body. As the omission of even a single alphabet letter prevents the completion of a word, so does a deficiency of a single amino acid inhibit the proper formation of these chemical structures into new proteins. The new proteins are used for cellular reconstruction.

There are basically 22 amino acids. All are "essential" but the following must be obtained from your diet: arginine, histidine, isoleucine, leucine, lysine, methionine, phynylalanine, threonine, tryptophan, and valine. These may not be meaningful to you, but if you run across them in articles you now know they are not vitamins, enzymes, or something else. The body cannot make the essential amino acids, and nothing can substitute for them.

If there is a deficiency of one or more amino acids, the protein changes do not occur at all, or occur in proportion to the insufficiency of some amino acids. These tremendous variations in amino acid chain-like structures are partially responsible for the ability of one individual to eat a particular food without ill effects, while another person encounters severe allergic reactions.

PROPER DIGESTION CAN IMPROVE ALLERGIC REACTIONS!

The digestion of proteins starts in the stomach. The protein enzymes in the stomach are active only in an acid medium. Gastric glands secrete a large amount of **hydrochloric acid (HCL)** that activates the protein digestive enzyme **pepsin.** Pepsin splits proteins, and begins protein digestion. *The two functions of HCL are ...*

- *to promote pepsin activity; HCL deficiency is a frequent cause of allergies, and HCL in the stomach is affected by dehydration or over-hydration. So most people should drink water equal to one ounce for each two pounds of body weight daily! Water helps digestion when consumed 15-30 minutes before meals, and not during meals.*

- *to sterilize the stomach contents, called CHYME. A dog can raid a garbage can and not get sick, because he has a lot more HCL than humans.*

Protein breakdown is very complex; many enzymes act in different stages of digestion. No single enzyme digests protein all the way to amino acids, the final stage, which is completed in the small intestine. *Proteins are split into three forms in the stomach in a time period based on the...*

- *amount of protein in the meal.*
- *size of the chunks of protein.*
- *amount of fat in the meal (1 1/2 - 4 hrs. or longer).*

Acid chyme empties into the duodenum (the first part of the small intestine), then is alkalized by sodium bicarbonate from the pancreas. It mixes with intestinal bacteria, enzymes from the pancreas and small intestine, to continue the digestion of starches, fats, and proteins. The health of the small intestine is greatly affected by good bacteria, Candida yeast, parasites, pH balance, and water.

The common factor of any symptom of poor digestion, heartburn, stomach distress or inflammation is the change initiated by dehydration. Symptoms like nausea, or a dislike of water will change as you become more hydrated. Water means distilled or filtered water; it does not mean regular tea, coffee, alcohol, or caffeine containing beverages. They contain dehydrating agents, and get rid of the water they are dissolve in, plus some from the body.

129

A preference for soda and juice will reduce the urge to drink plain water, even when the soda or juice is not available. You end up feeding Candida yeast and parasites with the extra sugar, and still produce dehydrated cells.

Do not drink in large amounts at one time, thinking you can undo the damage of many months or years of dehydration by excessive intake in a few days. **You need to drink a little at a time over the whole day for months, before full hydration of the body is achieved.** *Divide your day into blocks of time starting when you get up in the morning until about 8-9 PM. The total amount of water for the day should be evenly divided during those blocks of time. For example: You need to drink ten glasses of water daily, and you get up at 6 AM. You should have one quart in by 12 Noon, one quart in by 6 PM, and the other two glasses by 8-9 PM.*

FATS

Essentially, all fat is digested in the small intestine. The first stage is breaking up the fat globules by bile from the gallbladder. However, no bile is released from the gallbladder if you just eat fruit or vegetables. Bile is released only when fat enters the small intestine. If you do not have a gallbladder (one of the most performed surgeries in the U.S.), you have bile from the liver dripping continuously into the small intestine.

Some digestion of fat occurs from the small intestinal enzymes and healthy bacteria, but the most important action is from the pancreatic enzyme lipase. Fats are broken down to fatty acids and glycerol, before entering the blood to go to the liver.

Most absorption of nutrients occurs in the small intestine, as well as forming some vitamins like K, B1, B2, and B12. The job of the entire large intestine is to receive the fluid waste products of digestion, and store them until they are released from the body.

130

PANCREAS

The pancreas is a digestive organ in the abdomen that is located just below the stomach. It is responsible for producing digestive enzymes, alkalizing the small intestine, producing insulin to regulate blood sugar levels, and producing a special kind of alcohol (a deficiency can cause cold hands and feet, or general chilliness in all seasons). Pancreatic enzymes secreted include lipase, which digests fat, protease that digests proteins, and amylase, which digest starch molecules.

Stress, caffeine, alcohol, drugs, sugar, and refined food all *over* stimulate the pancreas, and eventually lead to its inability to produce either the acid-neutralizing bicarbonates, or enzymes. The health of the pancreas depends on the suggestions in this chapter (especially for a healthy liver), the good food discussed in the Nutrition chapter, and a colon cleanse two to three times a year. *Understanding that parasites can compromise the health of the pancreas is critical to your well being.*

[] [] [] [] [] []

MANY PEOPLE ARE OBLIVIOUS TO THE PROBLEMS OF DIGESTION, BECAUSE THEY THINK OF DIGESTION AS AN AUTOMATIC PROCESS THAT PROCEEDS WITH A CERTAIN DEGREE OF PERFECTION. **MAKING ASSUMPTIONS THAT THE FOOD YOU EAT IS ALWAYS DIGESTED, AND THAT THE DIGESTED FOOD IS ALWAYS ABSORBED, COULD BE THE FIRST WRONG STEP TOWARDS DEGENERATIVE HEALTH.**

We derive no value from undigested food. Undigested food in the digestive tract produces poisons that clog cells and lead to disease. Our society's first reaction is to treat burning sensations, heavy feeling after meals, nausea, vomiting, cramps, intestinal spasms, burping, poor appetite or constant hunger, sleepy after meals, and heartburn with modern medicine's *"new and improved"* products.

If your day is a continuous picnic, the stomach becomes an overloaded storage tank for undigested food. The outcome of this routine is fermentation, gas, mucus, and alcohol waste products that make you run to the corner drugstore for relief ... AGAIN AND AGAIN! Public opinion does not consider poor digestive symptoms a serious problem, because we have a wide selection of highly advertised, competitive over-the-counter digestive relief choices. You may feel better, which is the *MOST DANGEROUS* of all, because you are unaware of the collective damage of poisonous wastes. Treating only the symptoms, you would probably suffer these symptoms the rest of your life (which could be shortened unnecessarily). Or ... you could treat the **CAUSE** of the problem.

REMEMBER, YOU ARE NOT WHAT YOU EAT,
YOU ARE WHAT YOU DIGEST!!!

ARE YOU READY TO IMPROVE YOUR DIGESTION?

Some people take strict health suggestions and follow them to the letter. However, many people in this country are too busy living the American dream to do every healthy recommendation *all the time.* Those who want to be super-strict would find controversy in areas of this book. I am not trying to sway the thinking of those already dedicated. *I am trying to present a starting place for those whom never before thought they had to learn about the subject of digestion. I am trying to reach the multitude of people frustrated with disease, who have no idea how they got sick. I am trying to teach people that there is a much better way to treat chronic symptoms, then to **continuously treat chronic symptoms!** For those **beginners,** here are 10 important digestive guidelines:*

1. WHEN SHOULD YOU EAT YOUR PROTEIN AND WHEN SHOULD YOU EAT YOUR SALAD?

There are conflicting opinions; reading can produce total confusion. In Europe, they eat their salad after the meal.

One opinion: *Every meal should begin with raw foods because you need enzymes of raw food to help digest other foods.*

Another opinion: *Protein foods need lots of HCL for proper digestion in the stomach. If the stomach is first filled with a large salad which does not require HCL for digestion, the protein eaten afterwards may not be digested well, because the diluted HCL is not strong enough to activate the protein enzymes.*

My recommended opinion: *A large salad should be eaten with protein, or after, but best not before protein. Raw foods do activate intestinal enzymes, but the digestion of protein begins in the stomach first.*

2. SIMPLE FOOD COMBINING

A strict version of this may need to be considered for people with severe digestive problems, or people recovering from a serious illness who need the best digestion.   Correct food-combining books best describe this guide to digestion. For most people, some principles discussed are too strict, and contradictory to our American way of eating (like no starchy and acidic foods together, means no more sandwiches). *There are, however, some basic principles that should be considered by everyone:*

-   *The simpler the meal, the better chance you have of digesting it.*

-   *Fats and proteins are not a good combination. A high-fat diet can inhibit the gastric juices and keep the food in the stomach hours longer, causing some foods to ferment. Eat a low-fat diet, but always remember you NEED essential fatty acids.*

- *Do not eat any form of sugar or sweet fruits with a meal containing normal protein intake (especially hard-to-digest animal protein). Sugar will ferment if delayed in the stomach. The exceptions are RAW pineapple and RAW papaya, which contain protein digesting enzymes. You may have a "special occasion" recipe that does not fit this rule. Both my sons want "strawberry lamb chops" for their birthday dinner.* **One donut will not destroy your health and one salad will not heal the body. It is what you do everyday that makes a difference.**

- *Desserts at the end of the meal combine poorly with almost every other part of the meal. They only complicate digestion. If you must have dessert, eat it alone one to two hours later.*

- *Fruits and vegetables are best eaten separately due to digestive interference in the same area of digestion...the small intestine. The one exception I make is mentioned in connection with blender drinks.*

- *The rule for best digestion when eating fruit is - EAT IT ALONE OR LEAVE IT ALONE! Melons, especially, will decompose quickly if held up in an acidic stomach, and will ferment.*

3. EAT SMALL MEALS, EAT SLOWLY, DRINK WATER BEFORE MEALS, AND CHEW FOOD EXTREMELY WELL!

"Drink your solids, and chew your liquids." If you chew well, eat small amounts, drink ½-one cup of distilled or filtered water 15-30 minutes before eating to churn food for more effective enzyme action, and have enough HCL, about 98 percent of protein will be digested.

You may want to add apple cider vinegar to the water before meals to activate hydrochloric acid, and improve digestion (Check Resource References for book).

4. THE "NEVERS"

- Never chew gum on an empty stomach as it can fool the body, and causes digestive juices to flow. This can cause mild to acute stomach distress, or other digestive irritation in the small intestine.

- Never eat if not hungry, feverish, in pain, chilled, or emotionally upset (which greatly affects the digestive process). If you do eat; choose foods like blender drinks, raw fruit or vegetables … never heavy proteins.

- Never drink icy cold, or hot drinks with meals because sudden changes slow down the digestive process. Never drink a lot of liquid throughout the meal. This is not a good time to catch up on your daily intake of water. Flooding the digestive system with water during meals flushes out digestive enzymes and nutrients. Take supplements with the water just before meals.

5. PROVIDE A GOOD MEDIUM FOR HEALTHY INTESTINAL BACTERIA.

Foods such as soy yogurt (preferred over cultured milk products because of mucus symptoms, and high allergic potential of dairy), sauerkraut, soured vegetables, or sourdough bread, will help grow the healthy bacteria needed for good digestion.

It is very important to consider supplements that can assist in the balance and stability of the whole-interrelated digestive system. If you have taken antibiotics, eaten meat, dairy or poultry containing antibiotics, you should consider products (powder or vegicaps) that improve intestinal flora.

135

Your future animal products should be hormone and antibiotic free.

The diet you eat determines the bacteria in your intestines. A vegetarian will have bacteria that primarily consume carbohydrates. A high meat diet will produce bacteria that act on undigested protein. A high meat diet will also produce powerful chemical toxins like phenol, that is not neutralized by the liver, but passes unchanged into the bloodstream. *A person with chemical sensitivities would be wise to eat little or no red meat.*

6. ELIMINATE ALL "REFINED" CARBOHYDRATES SUCH AS SUGAR IN ANY FORM, REFINED CEREALS, AND WHITE FLOUR.

Refined foods add to constipation and can interfere with the health of the whole-interrelated system of digestion, elimination, liver and gall bladder. It is all right to be sociable, and have an occasional treat with "fun food." However, these foods rob your system of nutrients needed for normal body function, so it is best not to be TOO social.

The five worst things you can put into your body, other than straight poison and red meat, are "THE FIVE WHITES," according to the herbalist Ed Bashaw.

1. Refined white sugar and sugar substitutes
2. Refined white salt
3. Refined white flour
4. Refined white shortening
5. Pasteurized, homogenized white milk

7. REMEMBER THE BODY'S CIRCADIAN RHYTHM.

Nutrient "ingestion" and "digestion" is best from noon to 8 PM. Eating hard to digest food after 8 PM will interfere with the distribution, utilization, and rest cycle. An occasional late social situation will not be a major problem, but consistently eating late could adversely affect your health in hidden ways that spell "symptoms." People who routinely work and eat during unusual hours, notoriously struggle with health issues.

8. DO NOT TREAT CHRONIC ILLNESS LIKE ACUTE ILLNESS.

We may never know how all the drugs on the market affect our enzymes and digestive process. All drugs, because of their toxicity, induce a stress that interferes with digestion and absorption of nutrients **in some way.**

Find out WHY you are sick and eliminate the cause. DOCTORS ARE FREQUENTLY CRITICIZED FOR PRESCRIBING DRUGS, BUT DRUGS ARE NOT PRESCRIBED FOR PEOPLE WHO ARE HEALTHY! IF YOU TAKE BETTER CARE OF YOURSELF, YOU WILL NOT HAVE TO ASK DOCTORS TO MAKE YOU WELL! Consider less traumatic ways to deal with symptoms, such as herbs, whole food supplements, environmental protection with antioxidants, water, protection from electromagnetic polluted frequencies, homeopathy, exercise, and improved nutritional choices. Living by the following **"LAWS" OF WELLNESS** may protect your health so you do not experience chronic illness:

(1) WATER: Drink at least eight glasses of distilled or filtered water per day. For most people the rule is one ounce per two pounds of body weight, unless medically restricted. If you have cold, flu, or pain symptoms, drink several extra glasses of water for two days. A cold is your body stating you are struggling with a build-up of toxic wastes. The flu is your body stating you are losing the battle dealing with toxic wastes. These too frequently experienced illnesses are considered inconveniences, rather than body language telling us we are unhealthy.

(2) TRACE MINERALS: Unless you eat only organic fruits and vegetables, and have perfect hydration and

137

*digestion, you need a trace mineral supplement. Trace
minerals act as catalysts in every activity of your body
every second of your life. This is too important to not
know the quality, and absorbability of what you are
buying.*

*You should acquaint yourself with the inorganic
minerals, available in the Bio-Plasma cell salts, that act
as electrical energy in your body. THE BIOCHEMIC
HANDBOOK lists ways to assist the body to heal itself;
cell salts are discussed later in this chapter.*

*(3) **ESSENTIAL FATTY ACIDS:** Consider two teaspoons
of Flaxseed oil or one tablespoon of ground Flax seeds
twice a day with some sulfurated protein like soy, or
whole wheat bread. Other essential fatty acid products
include Black Currant Seed oil (best for travel because it
breaks down slower without refrigeration than flaxseed
oil), Hemp oil, Borage oil, or Emu oil. Remember the
importance of essential fatty acids is to produce the
chemical prostaglandins that activate cellular activity.*

*(4) **pH BALANCE:** Test urine and saliva with pH paper a
MINIMUM of once a month. Fluids in your body have a*
proper pH balance; if out of balance, the fluid loses its
effectiveness. This is discussed in more detail later in
this chapter.

*(5) **CANDIDA YEAST OR PARASITE BALANCE**:
Recommend a lifetime version of the following diet to
control these two disease-producing organisms. Some
foods may be hard to eliminate socially, but should be
eliminated as much as possible at home.*

THESE FOODS ARE GREATLY REDUCED:

* fresh fruit one time daily only; no fruit juices.

* *refined sugar; keep natural sugars like honey, maple syrup, molasses to a minimum.*

* *milk or dairy products (except occasional socially)*

* **refined** *grain (white flour, white rice, refined rye).*

THESE FOODS ARE EATEN IN MODERATION:

* **Whole** *grains: whole wheat, oats, rye, barley, spelt, brown rice, corn, millet, quinoa.*

* **Starchy** *vegetables: all beans, peas, soy, peanut, potato, sweet potato, buckwheat, and squashes.*

THESE FOODS CAN BE EATEN AS DESIRED:

* ALL ANIMAL (beef, lamb, pork not recommended except occasionally), FOWL, EGG, FISH, SEAFOOD PROTEIN; OIL AND FATS; NUTS AND SEEDS; **AND ALL VEGETABLES NOT LISTED AS A** *STARCH DO NOT FEED CANDIDA YEAST OR PARASITES.*

(6) ELIMINATION: *Take an HERBAL laxative at bedtime if you do not have a good elimination by noon. Be more concerned about constipation, than the use of herbal laxatives.*

(7) EXERCISE: *Exercise allows the nutrients to get into the cells and the toxic wastes to get out of the cells, at a speed that allows the body to work at optimum performance. EXERCISE and WATER are the two main factors that keep the lymphatic system healthy, to eliminate toxic wastes from your blood. Oxygen from exercise and deep breathing activates intracellular energy. Your best "health friends" are exercise, water, and oxygen.*

You should deep breathe several times, six or more times daily. Breathe in through your nose and exhale deep from the diaphragm, not the mouth or throat. Your exhale should have a forced air sound to it deep from your lower lungs.

(8) STRESS MANAGEMENT: *Negative energy IS the greatest cause of illness ... and enthusiasm IS the most important predictor of wellness! Low self-esteem and low self-worth are epidemic in this country. Cellular health depends on the way you deal with stress management. THIS IS THE BOTTOM LINE. HEALTH DEALS WITH ALL LEVELS OF SPIRITUAL, MENTAL, EMOTIONAL, AND PHYSICAL AT THE SAME TIME! Read Chapter 1 again, and consider some of the recommended tapes and videos.*

IMPORTANT INFORMATION ...

Mercury vapors emitting from old mercury fillings may not be a "law" of wellness, but must be considered in any wellness program. Mercury is a poison, and Sam Ziff says in his book DENTISTRY WITHOUT MERCURY, *"Mercury poisoning is the biggest masquerader of our time. Dentists are not in a position to see the cause and effect relationship of the insertion of the mercury and the development of illness three to ten years later. Even the patient does not connect the illness to the original dental process."* THE NAME OF THE SYMPTOM, THE NAME OF THE DISEASE IS NOT YOUR PROBLEM!!! YOUR PROBLEM IS WHAT CAUSED THE SYMPTOM OR DISEASE.

The World Health Organization Environmental Health Criteria 118 document on inorganic mercury, confirms the escape of mercury vapor from amalgam dental fillings. Look for a dentist who has equipment to rate the level of mercury vapors emitted from your teeth. Be aware also that crowns can be placed over amalgam dental fillings. I could write a chapter on

140

this subject alone, but you owe it to yourself to get the facts from the experts who have written books on the subject.

Many dentists, like doctors do not support the cause of disease, and stick only to what they learned in their training. If you are struggling with any chronic health issue, and have *old amalgam dental fillings, or root canals,* I urge you to read books such as those listed in the Resource References. The success of your wellness effort could depend on **your** knowledge of those subjects.

9. DO NOT DRINK CHLORINATED OR FLUORIDATED WATER.

Chlorine destroys intestinal flora needed for good digestion. To eliminate chlorine, let the water set out overnight in a container, or bring to a boil and let it cool on its own. We do not always think of the chlorine in shower water, but you absorb 60 percent of what goes on your skin. Until you get a shower filter, take a short, warm shower with the bathroom door open. Breathing in all that hot, chlorine steam is not in your best health interest. Only use filters that take out chlorine, all heavy metal, parasites, and fluoride. Dr. Yiamouylannis, a Ph. D in Biochemistry is recognized as an international authority on the biological effects of fluoride. Industries stuck with fluoride as a waste product promoted it as a means of reducing tooth decay. It is quite evident that proper diet ... not fluoridation is necessary for good dental health. Fluoride as been proven harmful in court cases, and proven to cause genetic damage.

10. BE AWARE OF THE TIME RANGE FOR DIGESTION OF DIFFERENT FOODS:

Fruits	*1/2 hour*	
Herbs and vegetables	*1 hour*	
Seeds, nuts, grains	*2 hours*	
Fish	*2 hours*	
Fowl, lamb	*2-3 hours*	*(Heavy protein*
Beef	*3-5 hours*	*is best eaten*
Pork	*5-7+ hours*	*before 6PM)*

SOME SUPPLEMENTS THAT AID DIGESTION

1. **GARLIC** is nature's way of destroying harmful substances, and leaving beneficial organisms to assist in digestion.

2. **ALL NATURAL SUPERFOODS:** *The best supplements are not man made.* The body will always accept natural food better than synthetic fractions of nutrients, in a commercial supplement formulated in a chemist's lab. *All super-foods provide highly absorbable nutrients that allows the body to heal itself if possible, and work at optimum performance.* Products that contain alive super-foods consistently test excellent in my office on my biofeedback equipment. *Examples of "alive" super-foods are:*

    BEE POLLEN contains certain enzymes, which are essential catalysts in digestion. Bee pollen is capable of its own digestion, and aids digestion of other foods. It contains up to 30 percent protein, plus essential sugars, vitamins, minerals, and amino acids, all of which in its natural form is a nearly perfect food. As one of the richest foods in nature, it contains every basic ingredient needed to sustain life, so Bee Pollen is A POWERFUL NATURAL SUPPLEMENT.

    SPIRULINA PLANKTON is an algae that contains 70 percent protein, all essential amino acids, highest known source of B12, is a complete food similar to blue-green algae; both are excellent choices for total, natural nutritional, super food protection.

    BREWER'S YEAST is more than a treasure house of nutrients ... it is truly nature's wonder-food! Brewer's yeast varies based on how it is grown, and is discussed later in this chapter.

    BARLEY GREEN AND WHEAT GRASS juices are examples of the fast food of the future. Millions of people are now drinking grass for their health ... not the kind in the yard. Concentrated grass juice is dehydrated to a powder at low temperatures, allowing the enzymes to remain alive. There are no indigestible substances. All the nutrients, chlorophyll, enzymes, vitamins, and minerals are balanced by nature, easily assimilated, and absorbed directly through cell membranes in the mouth, throat, stomach and intestine.

3. **DIGESTIVE ENZYMES** available in health food stores, lessen the enzyme burden on your body, until your body becomes healthier. Your goal should be to balance the body so it functions correctly, and makes your own digestive enzymes. Enzymes are not destroyed during digestive chemical reactions, but they do break down and wear out. You can deplete your enzyme potential by living your life at a fast hectic pace. Since our lifestyles are often more stressful than we would like, it may be helpful to temporarily assist your body in enzyme activity. This is important if your urine or saliva pH is not normal. Digestive enzymes are abundant in alive food supplements, raw food, and food not heated over 130 degrees. I do not recommend digestive enzymes from beef or in beef capsules. Look for vegetarian products.

4. **HYDROCHLORIC ACID** tablets should be taken if saliva pH is too alkaline (generally above 6.4). Start with one tablet; add one extra tablet each meal until you feel warmth in your stomach. Next meal take the number of tablets that did not produce symptoms. You may consider apple cider vinegar before meals to stimulate stomach digestive juices; there are books available on this subject.

5. **MINERALS** are important catalysts in the utilization of proteins, fats and carbohydrates. Potassium is the mineral that opens up a tight digestive system. The humble prune is a powerhouse of potassium. Plumped with boiling water, they scrub your intestines. All diets should include mineral

supplementation, since commercial food may vary greatly in mineral content.

6. **B VITAMINS** are easily destroyed by the environment; in physical, emotional, and mental stress; and in processing or preparation of foods. B vitamins affect energy, digestion, nerves, growth, glandular output, emotions, circulation, immunity, and coordination. DO YOU GET THE MESSAGE? THIS IS NO TIME FOR REFINED, OVERCOOKED, AND PROCESSED FOODS!!! We must improve the *quality* of our diet first!!!

7. **ESSENTIAL FATTY ACIDS** in cold-pressed oils, whole grains, nuts, seeds, legumes, and supplements, break down to produce prostaglandins that act as chemical catalysts in body functions, including digestion.

8. **CAYENNE PEPPER** *is a miracle alkalizing food, because it is the best circulatory and digestion stimulating herb on earth.* Look for cayenne in the health food stores in vegicaps; always take with food. You may feel warmth in the stomach after taking cayenne, but the body should adjust after 1-2 weeks, and the sensation of warmth diminish.

[] [] [] [] [] []

JUICES THAT AID DIGESTION

FRESH, *RAW* **FRUIT JUICES** especially lemon, apple, and grape are the cleansers of the human body. Unfortunately, in our society we have become juice-aholics. That will do more harm than good, by providing enormous volumes of simple sugar to feed Candida yeast and parasites. We are also consuming *processed* juice that is pasteurized, so the enzymes are destroyed. Instead of helping, that puts a *stress* on the digestive system. If you want grape juice, you would be better off eating fresh grapes, and drinking a glass of water. Any tree-ripened fruit eaten fresh is a boost for the digestive system.

In chronic digestive problems, one-day juice fasts can help by giving the digestive organs time to rest and regenerate; more on this in the Elimination chapter. If you do fast with juice, you should dilute it ½ with water to reduce the concentration of simple sugar ingested at one time.

VEGETABLE JUICES are the regenerators and builders of the body. They contain **all the substances** needed for nourishing the body, providing the juices are **raw, fresh and preservative-free.** The best vegetables for the intestines are carrots, celery, cabbage, onion, garlic, and parsley.

[] [] [] [] [] []

VALUABLE HERBS NEXT ...

THE BASIC ASSUMPTION BEHIND NATURAL HEALING IS THAT THE HUMAN BODY IS LINKED TO THE PROPERTIES OF NATURAL ORGANIC SUBSTANCES.

Herbal remedies neutralize or eliminate from your body the harmful substances that impair its power to heal itself. You may not get a dramatic change in symptoms with herbs, like our society has learned to expect from drugs. Herbs gradually improve health as they influence the system to perform better in a more lasting way. *Herbs ...*

- feed, regulate, and cleanse the body naturally.

- give the body raw materials to do its own healing.

- are not as potentially dangerous as stronger drugs.

- should be part of any program in self-responsibility.

145

Looking back over the twentieth century there has been a revival of herbalism and natural healing, as the dangers in losing thousands of years of accumulated knowledge have become apparent. The twentieth century's rush for faster, more efficient, more convenient ways to do things has forgotten old ways. This rush *away* from nature has been termed "progress." Physicians have largely turned their medicine over to drug companies with their moneymaking patents. This takes the knowledge, and responsibility of SELF-HEALTH away from the individual.

POINTS TO REMEMBER WHEN TAKING HERBS:

1. Herbs frequently accelerate the action of each other, so the most effective way is to take them in combination.

2. Herbs are best taken WITH meals to prevent stomach upset.

3. Herbs are grown wild and contain maximum energy from sunlight and natural growth, providing valuable vitamins and minerals to supplement nutrition.

4. Herbs may be dried, so they could contain mold for the mold sensitive; it may explain why some people do not tolerate dried herbs in cooking, or herb teas.

5. Herbs are not all safe. Many contain powerful drug agents that have been used by medical doctors for years (i.e. digitalis). The average herb user is untrained, and habitual use can develop dangerous side effects (i.e. Ginseng Abuse Syndrome, which excites the nervous system). Herbal products are not labeled with side effects like drugs, so you should purchase a good herbal resource book. ROTATION is recommended after two to three bottles, both for possible side effects, and getting the benefits from a variety of excellent herbal choices.

6. Herbs in capsules other than vegicaps, may give someone sensitive to beef an allergic response.

DIGESTIVE HERBS TO DRINK - ginseng, *peppermint* and other mints, anise, chamomile, *licorice root*, comfrey (not regularly), fenugreek, *ginger root*, fennel seed, papaya, and cardamom. These herbal drinks at room temperature before meals may aid digestion.

DIGESTIVE HERBS FOR COOKING - thyme, rosemary, *ginger root*, papaya, garlic, dill, parsley, *cayenne*, sage caraway, and fennel seed.

DIGESTIVE HERBS AS SUPPLEMENTS - saw palmetto berries, catnip, slippery elm, goldenseal, myrrh gum, alfalfa (contains eight essential digestive enzymes - do not use if you are too alkaline), *licorice,* and *ginger.*

[] [] [] [] [] []

ACID-ALKALINE pH BALANCE

The Chinese knew about this 5,000 years ago, and called it yin-yang, or the balance of the life force. Modern medicine has almost forgotten it, and our society is paying an unnecessary toll for this lack of awareness.

Man's nature is governed by bio-electrical energy, which pulses as tides from acidity to alkalinity. You are most alkaline during rest, and the acid tide should dominate during the day. For proper body functions, a particular acid-alkaline balance must be maintained. *This balance is the regulation of hydrogen ion concentration in the body fluids:*

- *Hydrogen is an odorless, tasteless, colorless gas found in all organic compounds.*

- *pH stands for the potential (p) of the solution to attract Hydrogen ions (H); a pH of 7 is always neutral.*

- *a pH below 7 means high hydrogen ion concentration producing a too-acid system.*

147

- *a pH above 7 means low hydrogen ion concentration producing a too-alkaline system.*

In low resistance to chronic illness, your system may be too alkaline or too acid. The more alkaline your body pH is, the weaker your digestive juices become. If, for example, your urine is too acid, and your saliva is too alkaline, your body is very stressed.

In poor stress management, acidity dominates. An acid body pH means food must pass through the digestive system quickly to keep from burning the walls of the intestine. This means a decrease in absorption time for nutrients, and less energy for you. *If the urine and saliva pH is not normal, it does not matter what illness is present. Giving the illness a name does not correct the pH imbalance.* What does help is getting the pH back to a normal 6.4. This is a critical part of the "LAWS" OF WELLNESS. **You cannot achieve the degree of wellness you want without correct pH balance!** *Do not waste your time focusing on other possible solutions to your poor health, and ignore an imbalanced pH!*

We tend to think we are healthy unless we experience symptoms. Unfortunately, symptoms are the end process of body stress, not the beginning. If your pH is out of balance, YOU ARE PRODUCING THE STRESS THAT LEADS TO DISEASE. Circle the first day each month on your calendar to remind yourself to retest.

FOR HOME TESTING, TEST FOR pH AS FOLLOWS:

Saturate the pH paper with saliva, and another test strip with urine, first thing in the morning *before eating or drinking. Do not test any other time during the day!* Do not test pH before 6 AM, or after 8 AM. Repeat test for three days to average results. Normal urine pH should be 6.4, and saliva pH 6.5. Testing paper is available from some pharmacies, some mail order companies, or check with your local health food store.

HELP FOR pH

IF URINE OR SALIVA pH IS TOO ACID - 6.2 OR BELOW, CONSIDER THE FOLLOWING OPTIONS:

- *Take a neutral form of Vitamin C* like *calcium ascorbate, or Ester-C buffered. Do NOT take ascorbic acid!*

- *Eat alkaline forming food* listed in this chapter. *Be aware that excess fruits can encourage Candida yeast and parasite growth. Excess fruit can also put a stress on your thyroid or pancreas.*

- *Take Cell Salt Natrum Phosphate* as directed on bottle; *available in most health food stores.*

Health or illness is on the cellular level. The **"biochemic system of medicine"** is based primarily on the cell theory explained in *THE BIOCHEMIC HANDBOOK* published by Formur.

The workers of the cell - the 12 cell salts - are the inorganic constituents of the cell. If a deficiency occurs, a condition arises that produces a symptom. This theory of medicine states that every disease that affects the human race is due to a lack of one or more of these cell salts. To correct this disturbance, you need to know what salts are needed for what symptom, like diarrhea, stomach or leg cramps. This knowledge comes from chemistry, so the treatment of disease by supplying the needed cell salts is called BIOCHEMISTRY (bio meaning a combining form).

Tissue salts are safe at all times and cannot conflict with other treatments or medications. They are a natural part of your body chemistry. Cell salts replace what your body is missing, and are valuable options to drugs in chronic, or some acute conditions. I am not referring to drugs that are needed for critical body function, or may be life saving in emergencies.

- *No smoking*

- *Take digestive enzymes* with each meal based on bottle instructions. The amount you take depends on the size of the meal, amount of raw food, and fat content.

- *No caffeine except Green Tea.*

- *Stress increases acidity.* Become aware of the stressors in your life. Either accept them, or come up with a game plan to resolve them. Read Chapter 1 again. Poor stress management is a major cause of acidity, and must be addressed if other efforts to improve pH does not help.

- *Take chlorophyll supplements* that act as a balancing element for body chemistry.

- *One quart of vegetable blender drink daily* if you are too acidic!!

- *Use all natural Celtic Sea Salt* to neutralize the system.

- *Increase exercise,* because poor blood flow causes carbon dioxide accumulation, and decreases pH.

- *Neutralize any acute acidic condition* with baking soda, ½ teaspoon in four ounces of filtered or distilled water, and repeat in 30 minutes if necessary; or take two regular Alka-Seltzer (if aspirin tolerated). Acute acidic conditions include allergic reactions to food, medication, or bites of any kind.

IF URINE OR SALIVA pH IS TOO ALKALINE - 6.8 OR ABOVE, CONSIDER THE FOLLOWING OPTIONS:

- *Take ascorbic acid for your Vitamin C; switch to a buffered C or Ester-C when pH is 6.5.*

- *Eat acid forming food listed in this chapter.*

- *Take hydrochloric acid (HCL) tablets; or digestive enzymes.*

    When acids formed by foods which are not digesting correctly cause heartburn, and belching of acid stomach contents, we think it is an acid stomach condition. Actually, a lack of HCL can cause food to ferment and putrefy, causing unpleasant symptoms. Antacids help temporarily because they neutralize the fermentative acid, and what little hydrochloric acid may be present. This aggravates the condition by making the system even more alkaline. Check saliva pH before taking any antacid product. Do not take antacids if saliva pH is above 6.5 between 6 AM and 8 AM.

- *Improve elimination if transit time is not 12-18 hours. To test this, eat whole kernel corn, beets, or spinach for dinner. By noon the next day, you should see the corn, red or green color, depending on what you ate. Take herbal supplements, not commercial laxatives, if you do not eliminate by noon each day.*

- *Take Cell Salt Natrum Muriaticum, according to bottle directions.*

The natural ratio in a normal, healthy body is about four parts alkaline to one part acid. This ideal ratio maintained by your diet provides a strong resistance to disease; it is called the **RULE OF 80/20.** This rule means 80 percent of your food should be *alkaline forming*, and 20 percent should be *acid*

151

forming. In the typical American disease producing diet, the ratio is reversed.

ACID AND ALKALINE FOODS

There are two types of acid and alkaline foods. Acid and alkaline food means how much acidity or alkalinity the food contains in nature.

Foods react in the body according to digestion, so acid forming or alkaline forming means the changes foods undergo after being digested. What is important to your health is the acid or alkaline FORMING state of foods.

Acid *Forming* Foods	Alkaline *Forming* Foods
Eggs	Unrefined salt
Beef	Sprouted grains
Pork	All vegetables
Lamb	Fruits (expect cranberry, plums,
Chicken	prunes, blueberries)
Fish/Seafood	Herbal teas
Milk/all dairy products	Cooking herbs and spices
Goat's milk	All fresh beans
Grains (except millet,	Untreated oils
Quinoa, Amaranth)	Raw apple cider vinegar
Nuts (except almonds)	Sweet brown rice vinegar
Dried beans	Yeast
(except soybean)	Raw honey, Sucanat, Brown
Peanuts	rice syrup
Processed sugar, artificial	
sweeteners, maple syrup,	
molasses	
Alcoholic beverages	
Peanuts	
Coffee, black tea	
Carbonated beverages	

[] [] [] [] [] []

152

THE BASIC CAUSE OF DISEASE IS AN IMBALANCE IN YOUR BODY CHEMISTRY, which leads to an imbalance in what is called the Autonomic Nervous System. This system regulates all the parts of the body you do not control consciously … blood, circulation, digestion, and glands.

TWO BRANCHES OF THE AUTONOMIC NERVOUS SYSTEM:

- Sympathetic branch, *activated by acidity and calcium.*
- Parasympathetic branch, *activated by alkalinity and potassium.*

All organs and tissues have both. One branch excites the organ or tissue, and the other branch slows it down; they regulate each other like a gas pedal and a brake pedal. When the body is working normally, both branches are in balance, and organs function properly because neither branch dominates. *WHEN ONE BRANCH IS DOMINANT THEN THE OTHER BRANCH IS WEAK.*

THE SYMPATHETIC NERVOUS SYSTEM SPEEDS UP THE FUNCTION OF THE:

- heart	*- thyroid*	*- ovaries*
- adrenal	*- pituitary*	*- testes*

THE PARASYMPATHETIC NERVOUS SYSTEM SPEEDS UP THE FUNCTION OF THE:

- pancreas	*- intestines*	*- digestive system*
- liver	*- stomach*	*- colon*

One example of what happens when these two systems are imbalanced:

When your parasympathetic system dominates (pH too alkaline), potassium is INCREASED in the cells and calcium LEAVES your cells. Calcium is necessary for cell strength, so the membranes weaken and become too porous. This allows allergens to irritate or even penetrate the cells. The result provokes an allergenic response as the cells produce excess histamine in defense. In an effort to get rid of the excess histamine, the cells discharge it through the weakened cell membrane. This action irritates the connective tissues, and dilates the blood vessels. Fluids leak from tissues and blood vessels, causing swelling and inflammation that produce pain, and the reactions you call allergy symptoms.

WITH SO MUCH STRESS IN OUR SOCIETY, MANY PEOPLE PRESSURE THEIR SYMPATHETIC SYSTEM TO EXHAUSTION. THE DOMINANT PARASYMPATHETIC SYSTEM TAKES OVER, AND SERIOUS ILLNESS AND DEGENERATIVE DISEASE CAN DEVELOP. AS IT TOO BECOMES EXHAUSTED, CHRONIC ILLNESS BECOMES A WAY OF LIFE … AND DEATH. We need to stop blaming heredity for our poor health. A person can improve hereditary tendencies living by the "LAWS" OF WELLNESS.

WHAT FACTORS AFFECT NORMAL FUNCTION OF THE SYMPATHETIC SYSTEM?

- **Prolonged stress** over stimulates this system, and will eventually weaken the sympathetic system.

- **Poor calcium metabolism** discussed in Chapter 5.

- **Acid forming foods consumed in excess** will over stimulate the system, and eventually weaken it.

- **Too much Vitamin D** can cause excess calcium assimilation, so watch the amount of fortified food you eat. This, again, will first over stimulate the system, and then weaken the system.

- **Weakened sympathetic nervous system from birth;** we are producing less healthy children than our forefathers.

- **Low exercise** causes carbon dioxide accumulation, and that can decrease pH.

- **A deficiency in alkaline minerals** such as organic sodium, potassium, calcium, magnesium, manganese, and iron. *This is no time for refined and processed foods.*

WHAT FACTORS AFFECT NORMAL FUNCTION OF THE PARASYMPATHETIC SYSTEM?

- **Excessive amounts** of some common foods like avocado, bananas, grapes, tomatoes, broccoli, beets, cabbage, carrots, celery, garlic, all lettuce, potatoes, beans, peas, green beans, and parsley contain high levels of potassium and can over stimulate this system. Too many people eat the same foods over and over again. **MODERATION AND ROTATION IN ALL FOODS IS RECOMMENDED!**

- **Constipation** produces an alkalizing substance called "guanidine," which in excess can alkalize the cells and cause the parasympathetic system to become dominant. Both a too acid and a too alkaline system will benefit from a cleansing program. You are constipated if you do not have a good bowel elimination before noon.

- **Too much junk food, and poorly digested red meat and dairy**, puts an overload on the kidneys, so they are less effective in controlling proper ratios of acid-alkaline balance in the body.

- **Poor calcium absorption** to stimulate the sympathetic system. There are many things that can interfere with calcium utilization. *You must have good digestion, absorption, and metabolism.*

- **Excessive use of antacids** ... check your pH! If you continue to treat the symptoms ... you will have to *continue* to treat the symptoms! *Suppressing poor digestive symptoms without improving digestion, can only produce further ill health in the future.*

- **Deficiency of chloride ions caused by prolonged salt restricted diet.** *ABNORMAL RESTRICTIVE DIETS WILL NOT MAKE A BALANCED, HEALTHY BODY!*

- **A lack of hydrochloric acid in the stomach**; low zinc levels reduce stimulation of stomach cells to produce HCL, and water is needed to release HCL.

- **Poor liver function** reduces absorption of Vitamins A and E needed for strong cell membranes. Taking these supplements without a healthy liver can produce less than desired results. Without strong cell membranes, alkalinity is more likely to occur.

[] [] [] [] [] []

YOU NEED TO …
LEARN TO LOVE YOUR LIVER

The "liver" is very aptly called liv-er; without it, life is impossible. *The liver almost never feels painful, yet a person with a healthy liver is a rare exception because of…*

- bad diet choices typical in our society.

- multiple addictive habits.

- chemicals in our food and our environment.

- less healthy children being born each generation, means the liver can be overworked at birth.

One cannot live long without their heart, brain, kidney or pancreas, yet it is proper liver function, which prevents these organs from becoming diseased. It is the largest single organ of the body, surpassed by none in the importance of its various activities. It has great capacity to regenerate if deterioration is not extensive, and is the only organ that will regenerate itself if part of it is cut away. It is a magnificent piece of creativity, responsible for over 560 tremendously important functions.

Disease is largely due to 2 changes in the body:

- *nutritional deficiencies*
- *toxic build-up*

A poor functioning liver is involved in both of these problems, so the entire body will be affected.

SOME ACTIVITIES PERFORMED BY THE LIVER:

- Chemicals in your food, drugs, and environment pass through the liver and are either converted into forms usable by the body, or detoxified and discharged into the bile.

   *Your responsibility is to minimize chemicals in your food and environment, **so the liver does not have to work so hard**. It takes body energy and nutrients BORROWED from normal body functions to eliminate chemicals you could choose not to be exposed to, use, or consume.*

157

- Enzymes are made in the liver, which aid digestion. Enzymes supply the raw materials used by organs, glands, and tissues. This is a *BIG JOB*, and yet your liver does it every day of your life. WITHOUT ENZYMES, LIFE WOULD BE IMPOSSIBLE! THE LIVER CANNOT MAKE OVER ONE THOUSAND ENZYMES ON JUNK FOOD!!! ***THINK ABOUT THE REAL FOOD VALUE OF WHAT YOU EAT AND DRINK!!!***

- Antibodies to protect against infectious diseases are produced in the liver.

- The clotting factor which keeps you from bleeding to death is an appreciated liver function.

- The building blocks of proteins - amino acids - are converted in the liver into usable nutrients.

- Normal blood glucose concentration is maintained in the liver by taking excess glucose from the blood, storing it as glycogen, and restoring it to the blood as glucose when needed.

- Conversion of carbohydrates and proteins into sugar and fat when they are needed for energy, or eaten in excess.

- An overactive liver can cause homeothermic imbalance producing heat intolerance, or an underactive liver causing intolerance to cold. Think about the liver if you cannot handle temperature changes.

- Cholesterol is formed in the liver, of which 80 percent is converted into bile salts. New amounts of bile are formed in the liver to replace the amount lost through elimination. Constipation can really mess up this process of eliminating excess cholesterol. The bile acid that is not eliminated is reabsorbed back into the liver, and re-circulated instead of making new bile acid. Excess cholesterol that should be in new bile acid is now circulated in the blood, and that can lead to high cholesterol levels in the bloodstream.

BILE SALTS HAVE FOUR MAIN FUNCTIONS:

1. *They lubricate the intestines to aid in elimination.*

2. *They emulsify, or break up, the fat globules into minute size.*

3. *They help in absorption of fatty acids, cholesterol and other lipids from the intestinal tract.*

4. *They regularize the proper balance between the healthy intestinal bacteria and the unhealthy micro-organisms, like parasites or worms. Poor bile acid production creates a disorder in the intestinal flora, causing some species to disappear and others to multiply.*

- Lecithin is produced by the liver to dissolve fats within itself or in the bloodstream, supports healthy skin, feeds muscles and brain.

- Forms urea to remove ammonia from the body fluids. Without it, extreme toxic conditions develop rapidly.

- Excretes bilirubin, which is the end product of hemoglobin decomposition when blood cells have lived out their life; the liver stores iron from which new blood cells are made.

Iron stored in the liver will remain there, unless there is enough Vitamin C in the bloodstream, copper in the hemoglobin, Vitamin E in the tissues, essential fatty acids, cobalt, and 19 different amino acids. The "Prima Donna" iron particle will collect in the liver with inadequate B6 (which itself needs enough hydrochloric acid to be assimilated). SO MUCH FOR ONE IRON PILL SOLVING

159

YOUR IRON DEFICIENCY!!! A better way to deal with iron deficiency is to improve your diet, balance your pH for better absorption of nutrients, and take alive food supplements. If you need extra iron, consider liquid herbal iron products from the health food store.

- Stores fat soluble vitamins A, D, E, F and K; also stores, copper, some trace minerals and B vitamins.

- Inactivates hormones when they are no longer needed. Very important considering the increase in hormone related cancers, like breast and prostate cancer.

REDUCED FUNCTIONING IN ANY OF THESE AREAS LEADS TO CONDITIONS THAT CAN DEGENERATE ANY PART OF YOUR BODY.

[] [] [] [] [] []

THE LIVER ACTS AS A FILTER FOR THE REMOVAL OF TOXINS AND NUTRIENTS BETWEEN IT AND THE HEART:

The liver has a double circulation system, meaning that it receives blood from both the veins (carry blood towards the heart), and the arteries (carry blood away from the heart). If the body had no way of filtering out chemicals or impurities, they would keep circulating indefinitely, causing permanent change and eventually death. Fortunately, we have several systems for removing them as back up for the liver ... intestines, lungs, kidneys, and skin. BUT THE LIVER IS THE GREATEST PURIFIER OF THEM ALL.

[] [] [] [] [] []

PROBLEMS FROM A MALFUNCTIONING LIVER:

- **POOR DIGESTION** includes a red nose, chronic or acute nausea, gas, bloating, belching, anal itching due to the irritation from the heat of fermentation, heartburn, chills, fatigue, headache, sleepy after meals, and a general sluggish feeling.

- **POOR ELIMINATION** could be the root of headaches, low back pain, intestinal spasms, cramps, fatigue, or irritability.

- **URINARY PROBLEMS** that cause you to get up at night can be a sign of food allergies. Liver problems are always a part of allergies.

- **ABNORMAL INTESTINAL ORGANISMS** like worms, parasites, or Candida yeast.

- **INTESTINAL INFLAMMATION** like appendicitis, colitis, diverticulitis.

- **STOMACH ULCER** is always preceded by a liver disorder; food allergies need to be evaluated (especially milk, wheat, or gluten grains). *IT IS VERY IMPORTANT TO EVALUATE WATER INTAKE!*

- **MALNUTRITION** develops because food is not properly utilized by the body. It is not enough to take supplements and eat right. The organs involved with the body mechanics for utilization of nutrients must be healthy. *ANY PROBLEM DUE TO A LACK OF NUTRIENTS GOES BACK TO THE LIVER. ONLY HALF THE NORMAL AMOUNT OF BILE IS PRODUCED BY THE UNHEALTHY LIVER CAUSING CHRONIC POOR DIGESTION.* Vitamin C plays a vital role in the production of bile acid.

- **OVERWEIGHT OR UNDERWEIGHT** is at least partly due to insufficient enzymes to correctly transform and utilize food; or it can be due to low intracellular energy. To activate intracellular energy you need magnesium; normal iron levels to carry oxygen, and enough Vitamin C to release iron from the liver. You also need normal body pH, and hydration for proper digestion, so the liver can make Q10 to activate intracellular energy. Weight control is a lot more complicated than just dieting to lose weight, or overeating to gain weight.

  Overweight can be a sign of dehydration, since the sensation of thirst and hunger are generated simultaneously in the brain. We assume the urge is to need food, when the body may actually be calling for **WATER**. By drinking water before eating, you may find your "hunger" satisfied.

- **ANEMIA** from a malfunctioning liver leading to destruction of red cells, both old and new.

- **DIABETES** can develop from a sugar excess in the blood and urine, if the liver cannot handle the sugar coming from the intestines. The pancreas cannot do its job without enzymes from the liver.

- **SWELLING of legs and ankles** relate to liver function (also kidney and heart, which the liver keeps healthy).

- **SKIN DISEASES** produced from toxic substances not neutralized by the liver like acne, rashes, and liver spots. Candida yeast, parasites, bacteria, food allergies, and heavy metal toxicity can contribute to skin symptoms ... and unhealthy liver function is always involved.

- **GLANDULAR IMBALANCE** at menopause, and during the menstrual period, can be a problem from a malfunctioning liver. The liver is responsible for detoxifying accumulated female hormones that can produce sore breasts, and other symptoms associated with female menses.

- **NERVOUS SYSTEM DISORDERS** from retained toxic wastes can affect all systems. The liver must keep up with the toxic load in the body. *YOU CAN DO A LOT TO REDUCE TOXIC OVERLOAD BY REDUCING CHEMICAL EXPOSURES, AND MAKING BETTER FOOD CHOICES.*

- **OVERLOADED LYMPHATIC SYSTEM** is caused when the liver can no longer neutralize all the toxins that circulate in the blood. When blood leakage is filtered by the lymph system, organs like the tonsils can get overloaded and inflamed. A tonsillectomy will not solve your *long-term* health problems, if the reason for your lymphatic system congestion is not resolved!!!

- **REDUCED ABSORPTION OF FAT SOLUBLE VITAMINS A, D, E, F, AND K** due to poor bile production … remember to take your Vitamin C.

- **EAR PROBLEMS** can be due to general congestion of the body. This toxic overload can contribute to local chaos that encourages Candida yeast, parasites, viruses, and bacterial involvement. Ringing in the ears may need a liver evaluation.

- **SINUS PROBLEMS, HEAD COLDS,** AND **CHRONIC RESPIRATORY PROBLEMS** are a waste of time to treat symptomatically, and not deal with the liver condition. Colds are more prevalent in the winter when the liver is overworked from a heavier diet, and less exercise.

- **MENTAL DISTURBANCES** can occur from toxicity not correctly eliminated by the liver. The brain is 85-90 percent water. Sometimes mental health can be improved with **correct water intake alone.**

- **TENDENCY TO HEMORRHAGE** since the liver produces fibrinogen, an aid to blood coagulation.

163

- **CANCER** always includes poor liver function as part of the problem.

- **STERILITY AND IMPOTENCE** relate to the quality of our hormone production, from the nutrients our bodies receive from the liver.

- **HYPERTENSION** has liver congestion as its most common cause.

   All the blood in the body flows through the liver, both to pick up nutrients which the liver stores, and for detoxification. If the liver is congested with toxins or chemicals, overridden with fatty degeneration, or has become hardened from alcohol abuse, a back pressure builds up that can be reflected in the whole body circulation as hypertension.
   The Resin-Angiotension (RA) system is the pivotal mechanism for restoring body fluid balance. This system is activated when water is diminished, and tightens the vascular system in a way that can be measured and called hypertension. MANY PEOPLE WHO DRINK THEIR CORRECT AMOUNT OF WATER DAILY AND FOLLOW THE OTHER LAWS OF WELLNESS, NO LONGER SUFFER FROM HYPERTENSION.

- **HEPATITIS, OR LIVER INFLAMMATION** may result from a sick and weak functioning liver due to incorrect hydration, digestion or elimination problems, drugs, or chemicals, Candida yeast or parasite overgrowth, bacteria or viruses, electromagnetic polluted frequencies, or poor stress management. A suppresed immune system **must** be addressed to control liver disease. Hydration, pH balance, diet, and digestion **must** be addressed to control liver disease. Exercise and stress management **must** be addressed to control liver disease.

THE LIST OF PROBLEMS GOES ON WITH ARTHRITIS, ALLERGIES, ANEMIA, BODY ODOR, AND FATIGUE. MANY SYMPTOMS RESPOND TO LIVER DETOXIFICATION, WATER TO HYDRATE THE BODY, AND DAILY EXERCISE TO MOVE THE LYMPHATIC SYSTEM.

[] [] [] [] [] []

OUR KNOWLEDGE OF THE LIVER MUST BE EXPANDED AS OUR TECHNOLOGICAL AGE WITH ALL OUR MODERN EXPOSURE TO NEGATIVE ELECTROMAGNETIC FREQUENCIES, TO CHEMICALS, DRUGS, NUTRITIONALLY INFERIOR FOOD, AND ADDICTIVE HABITS CONTINUES TO GROW. Now that you know WHY you should "love your liver," let's talk about ways to protect the health of this hard-working, valuable organ. Besides the recommendations listed, health food store personnel can assist you in selecting homeopathic and herbal products to support liver health. Consult with your attending physician if you question any recommendation due to your medical history.

SOME FOODS THAT ARE BAD FOR THE LIVER:

- **The basic American diet** can produce liver damage!!!

- **Regular alcohol consumption** contributes to general toxicity.

- **Rancid oils** are very hard on the liver. Keep cold-pressed oils, whole grain flour or whole grain bread, and nut butters in the refrigerator; coffee, extra whole grain bread loaves, nuts and seeds in the freezer.

- **Red meat and animal fats** leave undigested waste products that are hard for the liver to neutralize. Excess protein depletes calcium reserves that can imbalance the pH, leading to poor digestion. Poor digestion will always put a stress on the liver.

- **Processed food, refined food, and food with chemical additives** provides minimal nutrition. Poor food choices must be replaced with food that can give the liver nutrients it needs to perform its many functions. JUNK FOOD, AND THE TYPICAL AMERICAN DIET IS NOT GOOD ENOUGH NUTRITION!!!

- **Margarine, processed oils, coffee, refined flour, refined sugar,** all make the liver deal with chemicals and/or acidity, without getting quality nutritional value!!!

- **Pasteurized milk** is poorly digested by adults; any undigested food is hard on the liver.

[] [] [] [] [] []

SOME CHOICES THAT ARE BAD FOR THE LIVER:

- **Excess fatigue**, both physical and mental, produces toxins that may tax the liver beyond endurance.

- **Overcooked food** destroys nutrients and enzymes, requiring the liver to work harder in the digestive process.

- **Overeating** strains the liver because of the effort to get rid of toxins resulting from poor digestion.

- **Lack of exercise** reduces the ability of the lungs and skin to help the liver in the elimination of toxins.

- **Not enough WATER** reduces the lymphatic system, and the kidneys ability to help the liver in the elimination of toxins.

- **Constipation** seriously reduces the bowel's ability to help the liver in the elimination of toxins.

166

- **Ingested or inhaled chemicals** are hard on the liver. New homes or offices, hobbies, and job choices may not be something that you can, or want to change. *YOU MUST, HOWEVER, BE AWARE OF THE DAMAGING EFFECT ON YOUR LIVER, AND MAKE EFFORTS TO HELP IT IN THE STRUGGLE, WITH HEALTHY FOOD, WHOLE FOOD SUPPLEMENTS, FILTERED WATER, ANTIOXIDANT SUPPLEMENTS, AND EXERCISE.* You can survive better in today's chemical exposures if you practice the "laws" of wellness.

- **Stress, caffeine, tobacco, and social drugs** make the liver produce enormous elements of defense.

- **Prescription drugs** should be for acute situations, life-saving situations, or body functions (like insulin or thyroid). Always find out WHY you have the problem so you can treat the CAUSE and not just the symptoms. When you have chronic problems, **THE NAME OF THE SYMPTOM, THE NAME OF THE DISEASE IS NOT YOUR PROBLEM ... YOUR PROBLEM IS WHY YOU GOT THE SYMPTOM OR DISEASE.** Treating the symptoms will **NEVER** treat the cause!

THE LIVER WORKS VERY HARD FOR YOU, AND WAS NOT INTENDED TO PUT UP WITH SMOKING; EXCESSIVE ALCOHOL; EIGHT TO TEN POUNDS OF CHEMICALS PER YEAR; SOCIAL AND PRESCRIPTION DRUGS; HIGH SUGAR, HIGH FAT, REFINED AND PROCESSED DEAD FOOD!!! TO OUR GREAT FORTUNE THE LIVER HAS A TREMENDOUS CAPACITY TO RESTORE ITSELF TO NORMAL FUNCTION.

[] [] [] [] [] []

167

THE FOLLOWING RECOMMENDATIONS WILL HELP YOU IMPROVE THE HEALTH AND PERFORMANCE OF YOUR LIVER:

DIET

The liver, even with the best diet, has a tremendous job to do. Sometimes the liver gets clogged up with body wastes, resulting from over-consumption of the "dead" foods, which are continually being eaten. Instead of treating the symptoms of toxic build-up (like a headache), the sensible thing to do is to lighten the work of the liver. This is best done by eating only such foods as can be easily digested, and will have minimal end wastes to be cleansed from the system. *This is called a MUCUSLESS DIET. The strict version ELIMINATES...*

- *all processed foods, refined sugar and flour.*

- *use of refined commercial table salt.*

- *eggs.*

- *milk and all dairy products.*

- *all red meat (beef, pork, lamb, buffalo, deer, elk).*

- *any grain that is heated over 130 degrees is mucus-forming.*

ALLOWED FOODS INCLUDE...

- *all FRESH fruits and vegetables.*

- *all fish, seafood, rabbit, hormone and antibiotic-free chicken and turkey.*

- *all nuts and seeds (raw or dry roasted).*

168

-   *all cold-pressed oils.*

-   *all herbs and spices.*

-   *all natural sugars like honey, molasses, maple
    sugar.*

-   *sun-evaporated or solar seasalt, or Celtic salt.*

-   *all sprouted or whole grains, such as stone ground
    whole wheat, oats, rye, barley, spelt, brown rice,
    corn, and millet. NOTE: Cooked whole grains are
    mucus forming, but provide valuable fiber, B
    vitamins and other nutrients. Unless a person is
    trying to eliminate a lot of mucus build-up from
    years of chronic sinus or respiratory problems,
    whole grains are allowed cooked, or as whole grain
    bread.*

-   *organic eggs needed for recipes are allowed, or as
    an occasional meal. The word is MODERATION.*

[] [] [] [] [] []

1, 2, OR 3 DAY CLEANSING

Dietary and supplement considerations will work better after
an initial liver cleansing program. A cleanse for three days is
best , but one or two days is better than nothing. You must
consume some oil (preferably olive oil) each day on a juice fast
to cleanse the gallbladder. *If for any reason you cannot fast just
on liquid, you may wish to add...*

-   *a few raw or dry roasted nuts or seeds.*

-   *any combination vegetable salad with homemade
    olive oil, lemon juice, and garlic salad dressing.*

169

- *skinned hormone and antibiotic-free white chicken meat, baked or broiled.*

Any recommendation should only be considered if you are drinking your tolerated amount of water each day, exercising seven days a week, and have a large bowel movement daily before noon. Your body needs to be hydrated, and elimination systems moving before you consider any cleansing option. This will reduce the discomfort from the cleansing process.

Apple or grape juice are both good cleansing choices, but may cause a problem if you have a Candida yeast or parasite overgrowth. In modern society, one degree or another of a Candida yeast and/or parasite problem may exist in most people, **so the safest choice is a lemon juice cleanse.**

*A simple lemon juice cleanse is alternating a tolerated solution of lemon and distilled or filtered water, with additional water for one, two, or three days. Your **total combined** liquid intake should be equal to one ounce for each two pounds of body weight (unless otherwise indicated). Put juice of three to six lemons in one quart of water, and rotate with plain water. Eat a mucusless diet.*

Another cleansing recommendation is:

Combine one tablespoon of extra virgin olive oil, a squeeze of fresh lemon juice, 1/2 teaspoon liquid garlic available in health food stores, and two tablespoons of Aloe Vera juice. Aloe of less quality than unrefined, whole leaf, and cold-pressed is not therapeutic enough. Start with 1/2 teaspoon of the mixture each morning, and slowly work up to consuming the full combination of ingredients each morning. Maintain that amount for two weeks. Only water or fresh fruit until noon; all food should be mucusless for one to two months.

[] [] [] [] [] []

A liver cleanse detoxifies, but also should include rebuilding the cells of the liver. Juices are the cleansers of the body, and vegetables are the rebuilders of the body. *Along with your cleanse include the following vegetables:*

Four times a day drink an eight ounce glass of any combination FRESH vegetable juice. Use a home juicer, blend a variety of vegetables in a blender, or eat a large salad.

*Beets are a powerful cleanser and the best vegetable for the liver. NEVER DRINK BEET JUICE ALONE, OR IN LARGE QUANTITIES!! Start with 1/2 **small**, peeled raw beet as a part of every vegetable drink, or shredded on a salad; increase to one small beet daily as tolerated. Other vegetable choices should include celery, cabbage, kale, spinach, cucumbers, lettuce, carrots, tomatoes, or radishes.*

[] [] [] [] [] []

DURING EACH CLEANSE ...

- **Take a warm, relaxing bath or shower in the evening** before retiring. Showering is best if you have city water, because you can buy a filter to remove the chlorine. Nature eliminates poisons through the pores of the skin, which is a back-up system that reduces the stress on the liver.

  It is necessary to keep the skin clean and free of dead skin cells that clog the pores. Use a body brush daily to remove dead skin cells, that are better down your drain than in your bed. Microscopic mites feed off dead skin cells. Mite bites can cause allergic reactions, and stress the immune system ... so shower at night before going to bed.

- **IT IS VERY IMPORTANT THAT YOU HAVE A GOOD DAILY BOWEL MOVEMENT BEFORE NOON.** If not, consider a natural laxative at bedtime for one week, *before a colon cleanse.*

- During the cleanse, have **plenty of fresh air, rest, and water.** You may do stretching or mild exercise, but energy needs to go to internal cleansing. Strenuous exercise should be avoided until after the cleanse is over. If you have flu-like symptoms, reduce the cleansing choice, drink extra water, increase walking-type exercises, and resume when symptoms subside.

- **Practice positive affirmations and LAUGH!!** Laughing massages the liver and helps it function better … and, makes your day happier!

[] [] [] [] [] []

SOME FOODS THAT ARE GOOD FOR THE LIVER:

- **UNREFINED, COLD-PRESSED OLIVE OIL** IS THE OIL THAT BENEFITS THE LIVER MOST! Use as much as possible.

- **LEMON IS THE BEST FRUIT FOR THE LIVER,** and can replace vinegar in all seasonings. The liver and lemon are natural together. The secret health aide for most illnesses associated with a sluggish liver is the simple lemon.

- **BEETS ARE THE BEST VEGETABLE FOR THE LIVER.** *USE BEETS OFTEN!* They can be cooked, but even better shredded raw on salads or in blender drinks. You can buy beet crystals in some health food stores.

- **BREWER'S YEAST IS AN EXCELLENT ALL AROUND FOOD FOR THE LIVER.** It is one of the best natural sources of the entire B complex. It is a superb source of concentrated complete protein. It is rich in essential fatty acids, and trace minerals. It is the best nutritional source of Chromium in an organic compound known as GTF (Glucose Tolerance Factor) . GTF is essential for the production of functionally effective insulin. Lewis Laboratories Premium Brewer's Yeast is grown on Sugar Beets, and does not have the same negative taste of yeast grown on hops or grain. Since this Brewer's Yeast is not an active yeast, it need not have the same concerns for people with Candida yeast symptoms. Lewis Laboratories Brewer's Yeast is available in most health food stores, and many grocery stores. This Brewer's Yeast is delicious in chocolate, carob, or vanilla rice or soymilk.

- **A high fiber breakfast** helps start bile juices flowing to encourage the elimination that removes toxins from the system.

- **Garlic**'s power to detoxify bacteria in the intestines gives the liver rest. Garlic helps digestion, increases blood circulation through the liver, stimulates bile production, lowers blood fats, and is a general tonic.

- **All fresh berries** are excellent cleansing foods, and are one reason why people tend to be healthier during the summer months.

- **Parsley** should never be left to die on a restaurant platter. It stimulates the liver and helps to prevent gas and indigestion.

- **Nutrients the liver needs will be far more available if all foods were eaten in a fresh, unprocessed form, prepared and served as quickly as possible.** Supplements are a big temptation when a person does not feel well. However, no pharmaceutical preparation will ever replace the value of fresh food, supplements with phyto-chemicals derived from alive foods, and specific nutrients from all the natural super-foods. *THE BODY DOES KNOW THE DIFFERENCE!!!*

173

SOME HERBS THAT ARE GOOD FOR THE LIVER:

Note: Be aware the herbal supplements may be in beef capsules, and could be an allergic problem for some people.

- **Milk thistle** has become world famous as a liver protecting herb. Since herbs work best in combination, you should look for a liver formula containing milk thistle. Other herbs to look for, include: artichoke, Cascara Sagrada, Devil's Claw, Dong Quai, Feverfew, Schisandra, Cloves, and Turmeric.

- **Blessed thistle** aids the liver, digestive, and lymphatic systems. Most bitter herbs are good for the liver, like dandelion and goldenseal.

- **Alfalfa** contains chlorophyll for blood purification. Alfalfa is a good source of nutrients the liver needs, like B vitamins, Vitamin A, and Vitamin C. Do not take alfalfa if your pH is too alkaline.

- **Ginseng** is a fantastic tonic for the whole body, and *loves* the liver. It gives the liver energy to heal itself.

- **Licorice** is an ages-old healer and will soothe and help heal the liver. *It is one of complementary medicine's most powerful herbs.* It is very possible that the healing properties of this ancient root have only begun to be explored.

- **Herbal tea** for liver support includes any herb good for digestion, *as well as the following:*

    * **Chamomile** has long been known to help the interrelated system of liver/gallbladder by dissolving gallstones.

    * **Rosemary** is one of the most effective remedies for the liver.

*   **Sage** purifies the liver.

*   **Thyme** has antiseptic properties.

*   **Gingerroot** may help the liver lower cholesterol
    levels, and is an herb for all seasons. *Keep fresh
    gingerroot in the freezer, then chop about 1/2 inch
    off a peeled section. Steep in a cup of hot water for
    10 minutes, and strain ... delicious!*

REMEMBER, THE LIVER HAS AN AMAZING
CAPACITY TO REGENERATE ITSELF! A complete program
for liver renewal can take three months to one year. *You must
formulate a wellness program and consider it a lifetime
commitment. Why treat symptoms when a healthy liver is really
what the body needs.* **THE IMPORTANCE OF
MAINTAINING A STATE OF OPTIMUM HEALTH IN
THE LIVER, CANNOT BE OVER-EMPHASIZED!!!**

**THIS IS YOUR LIFE ...
IT IS NOT A REHEARSAL!**

[] [] [] [] [] []

Health is not just what you eat, digest, and eliminate
properly, it is also what you think! Regenerating the body is a
good time to think how **"YOUNG"** you are, rather than how old.
As your cells regenerate, you are literally a **"NEW"** person.
Think of all the newly born cells in your body ... no matter how
many years you have lived, there is new life being produced this
instant in your body!!! We forget the we are "newborns" our
whole life, and just like we nurture a baby, we need to nurture
our bodies.

Think new thoughts worthy of those new cells, because there
is automatic renewal in the world of cells, but not in the renewal
of the mind. YOU HAVE TO SEE TO IT THAT YOUR MIND
IN RENEWED!!!

175

THE BODY RENEWS ITSELF
ACCORDING TO THE MENTAL ATTITUDE IT HOLDS!

REMEMBER ...

HEALTH IS ON ALL LEVELS OF
SPIRITUAL, MENTAL, EMOTIONAL,
AND PHYSICAL.

[] [] [] [] [] []

Paul Meynell, editor of RESEARCH NUTRITION wrote:

The influence of heredity is minimal compared with that of environment. NUTRITION is an environmental factor. Defective nutrition is a major stress. Many reports from many sources indicate beyond doubt that acute diseases, organic diseases, and senile degeneration are all cellular diseases. The basic condition which makes cells vulnerable is inadequate nutrition. By training and social tradition, medicine has to do with DISEASE, and not with HEALTH. Health may be considered just another name for established and maintained BODY CHEMICAL BALANCE. When the balance is restored, through proper digestion of food, "symptoms" tend to disappear.

DIET IS WHAT WE EAT.
NUTRITION IS WHAT THE CELLS
ACTUALLY RECEIVE.

Our society favors the wrong kinds of liquid, overeating, eating of hard-to-digest proteins, eating wrong combinations, or

176

eating under physical and emotional stress. *WE CANNOT TAKE FOR GRANTED THAT THE PRESENT EATING PRACTICES OF MODERN TIMES ARE NORMAL. INSTEAD OF HEALTH, WHAT HAS BECOME NORMAL IS A SOCIETY OF SICK AND WEAKENED PEOPLE.*

Good digestion is your insurance plan for protecting health. Poor digestion and stress promotes toxicity that leads to disease. So, dear reader ... best read on and learn how to eliminate toxicity ...

CHAPTER 4

ELIMINATION

*"The natural healing force within us is
the greatest force in getting well."*

- Hippocrates, Father of Medicine

Information on symptoms arising primarily from intestinal toxemia have filled volumes. Every symptom does not arise from intestinal toxemia, but it is at the root of conditions more often than is suspected.

The basic premise of organic medicine is that the human body is self-curing when it functions properly. *Therefore, the duty of the physician is to promote normal function by:*

1. Caring for localized, or acute and crisis symptoms.

2. Restoring the body to its general biochemistry by:

    -   eliminating excess waste products from the blood and tissues.

    -   supplying nutrients to nourish tissue.

    -   restoring body harmony between interrelated systems like glandular/nervous, structural/muscular, and digestive/eliminative.

    -   promoting mental and emotional tranquility.

"The Doctor of the future will give no medicine but will interest their patients in the care of their body, their diet, and in the cause and prevention of disease."

- Thomas A. Edison

178

THAT IS HOLISTIC MEDICINE!

Unfortunately, modern medicine deals more with crisis medicine rather than restoring whole body health. Modern medicine too often does not resolve the "cause" of the problem. **Negative thoughts, body toxicity, cellular dehydration, and disharmony in the whole body continue to produce another crisis ... and another ... and another.**

"THERE IS ONLY ONE BASIC DISEASE - TOXEMIA, WHICH IS CELLULAR CONTAMINATION."

- Dr. Kurt Donsbach (a noted herbalist)

In most all cases of cellular malnutrition and decreased cellular health, you must FIRST have cellular contamination.

A HEALTHY HUMAN BEING HAS THOUSANDS OF WAYS TO DECREASE CELLULAR HEALTH:

1. Physical shock from serious acute illness or injury.

2. Emotional shock from loss of a loved one, family crisis, loss of financial stability, or serious change in general health.

3. Overeating, since too many people have the inclination to resist the LAWS OF HEALTH. We think overeating can be resolved by a pharmacy full of comfort aids.

4. Undereating from depression, shock, anorexia, and hopelessness.

5. Worry is a comfort zone when low self esteem prevents action.

6. Tension produces continued disharmony, because of the belief that, *"I can't be happy, and life is hard."*

179

These all interfere with digestion, elimination, absorption of nutrients, and put stress on the lymphatic system (discussed in the Internal Energy chapter). This sets the stage for the gradual accumulation of toxins. *These toxic poisons are composed of...*

- retained waste products not properly eliminated.

- toxic substances not detoxified by the liver or lymph system.

- absorbed toxic products of abnormal digestion.

- inhaled environmental chemicals, and ingested chemicals.

THESE OVERABUNDANT WASTES, SO TYPICAL IN OUR MODERN SOCIETY, DERAIL THE BLOODSTREAM'S DELIVERY TRAIN SO YOUR CELLS DO NOT GET THE NUTRIENTS THEY NEED ... PRODUCING CELLULAR MALNUTRITION.

[] [] [] [] [] []

FIVE THINGS THAT CAUSE SUB-HEALTH CONDITIONS:

1. Congenital deformity
2. Hereditary weakness
3. Organic injury
4. Cellular contamination
5. Nutritional deficiency

The first three represent five percent of all sub-health conditions. *THE LAST TWO REPRESENT 95 PERCENT OF ALL SUB-HEALTH CONDITIONS ... AND YOU ARE RESPONSIBLE FOR BOTH!*

Two of the most unrecognized sub-health conditions are Candida yeast and parasites. You should have in your home library, at least one book on Candida yeast, and one on parasites. *Books on these subjects are easy to find in health sections of bookstores, or health food stores that carry books.*

Candida yeast (a common yeast present in the human body) and parasites, are now being recognized as primary causes of health disorders throughout the human body. While Candidiasis has been named the "Twentieth Century Disease," parasites are the unrecognized "All Time Disease" promoters of the past, present and future.

We think Americans are too clean, too civilized, too well fed, and too well educated for parasites to be a serious problem...**WRONG!!!** *PARASITES KNOW NO NATIONAL BOUNDARIES, ARE OBLIVIOUS TO YOUR INCOME, YOUR NATIONALITY, YOUR AGE, AND YOUR BELIEFS.*

The world's population can be infected with parasites that can range from microscopic to 20 feet long. According to the Center for Disease Control, virtually every known parasitic disease has been diagnosed in the United States. Dr. Hulda Clark in her book, *THE CURE FOR ALL DISEASES*, describes parasites as the cause of both common and extraordinary diseases. *She says:*

> *"No matter how long and confusing the list of symptoms a person has, I am sure to find only two things wrong: they have in them pollutants and/or parasites."*

Symptoms of parasitic infections run a full range. All parasites weaken your immune system and invite serious illness and degenerative diseases, including that "not well" feeling. Since parasites disturb the balance in the intestines, many effects are symptoms like gas, constipation, diarrhea, bad breath, and irritable bowel syndrome. Examples of indirect symptoms that are a result of intestinal disturbance include joint pain, muscle pain (fibromyalgia syndrome), anemia, allergies, skin problems, nervousness, depression, sleep disturbances, fatigue, and sugar cravings. **PARASITES SHOULD BE SUSPECTED IF OTHER FORMS OF TREATMENT FOR GENERAL SYMPTOMS DO NOT HELP!!!**

YOU CAN GET PARASITES FROM ...

- inhaling dust containing organisms.
- shaking hands with an infected person; or sharing drinks.
- playing with your pet; being licked by pets.
- children who pick them up from friends at school.
- eating raw, unwashed vegetables (salad bars are big offenders).
- raw, rare and undercooked meat and fish and seafood.
- restaurant food handlers.
- intimate sexual contact; kissing (even on the cheek).
- international, social, or military travel.
- rural and urban water systems.
- careless diapering in day care centers.
- weakened intestinal flora after antibiotics, and immune suppressing drugs.
- imbalanced bowel flora, at least partly due to low bile acid production from the liver.

A MAJOR CONTRIBUTING FACTOR TO PARASITE OVERGROWTH IS A COLON CLOGGED AND IMPACTED, THAT PROVIDES A WARM AND WELL-FED BREEDING GROUND FOR THE EGGS OF WORMS AND OTHER PARASITES TO PROLIFERATE. THEY LOVE CONSTIPATION!!! A HEALTHY INTESTINE STARTS IN THE LIVER.

NATURAL PARASITE TREATMENTS

When you take any parasite product you might have some flu-like symptoms of die-off. It is best to take a colon cleanse to flush out any build-up of old fecal material. The parasites lay eggs in that environment. If you do not kill the eggs, you will continue to have new generations of parasites. *Parasite treatment programs include ...*

- green hulls of *Black Walnut* and *Wormwood* which are the best herbs to kill parasites; *cloves* are the best to kill parasite eggs. Health food stores carry products containing these herbs.

- herbs like pink root, male fern, senna, fennel, Tansy herb, Egyptian thorn, and Jerusalem Oak (also called American Wormseed).

- raw garlic or garlic juice, raw onions, figs, raw pineapple, and pumpkin seeds are powerful worm killers.

- cayenne pepper on your food; or take vegicaps one or two, three times a day. Cayenne should always be taken with food. The warmth in the stomach shows the action of cayenne, and if taken with food, symptoms should be reduced in several weeks.

- diatomaceous earth made from microscopic sea life that worms do not like.

- colonics just to clean out the colon. This is NOT recommended on a regular basis as *colonics also flush out good bacteria.*

- products and cleanses that improve liver function, since bile acid produced by the liver balances bowel flora, so parasites do not want to live there.

- diet low in simple carbohydrates like natural and refined sugar, fruit, fruit juices, milk and dairy products, and refined grains. You may not be able to restrict certain foods socially or while traveling, but most people *make or break their health at home. What you eat at home* *should follow as closely as possible the diet that does **not** feed microorganisms.*

DIET SPECIFIC FOR BOTH CANDIDA YEAST AND PARASITES IS WORTH REPEATING OVER AND OVER, UNTIL THE BASICS BECOME A WAY OF LIFE.

SIMPLE SUGARS TO ELIMINATE OR RESTRICT:

- Fresh fruit once, no more than twice a day. No fruit juices due to increased simple sugar content; a glass of orange juice contain four oranges. If you want orange juice, eat a fresh orange, and drink a glass of water!

- No refined sugar except for social occasions. Keep natural sugars like honey, maple syrup, and molasses to a minimum.

- No milk or dairy products due to milk sugar content; reserve dairy for social occasions only.

- No refined grains except social or occasional regular pasta. Whole grain pastas are nutritionally superior. Give them a chance ... many are as delicious as white refined pasta. Grocery stores are now carrying more unrefined foods.

STARCHY FOODS TO EAT IN MODERATION:

- Whole grains and starches break down to simple sugar slowly, and feed parasites (and Candida yeast) less than sugars, fruit, dairy, and refined grains.

  Whole grains include whole wheat, oats, whole rye, barley, spelt, brown rice, corn, and millet. Wheat, rye, and rice are the only grains that are refined.

Starchy vegetables include beans, peas, soy, peanut, potato, sweet potato, buckwheat, and squashes.

FOODS THAT DO NOT FEED PARASITES OR CANDIDA YEAST:

- Animal protein does not feed microorganisms, but red meat should not be consumed if there are digestive problems. Occasional social consumption of red meat in small amounts may not be a major problem. If consumed at home, animal protein should be hormone and antibiotic free. Fowl and egg should also be hormone and antibiotic free. Fish and seafood protein are best eaten in restaurants because they do not contain hormones and antibiotics. All protein selections should be rotated at home, so harder to digest meat selections are not eaten everyday.

- Oil and fats do not feed microorganisms. Butter should be organic; oils should be *cold-pressed*.

- Nuts and seeds do not feed microorganisms. Shelled nuts and seeds should be kept in the freezer until needed. Because of the high fat content, they do not freeze, and can be eaten right from the freezer. Do not let nuts or seeds sit out in a dish all day, because they *do turn rancid*.

- All vegetables not listed as a starch do not feed microorganisms. Eat yellow, orange, and dark green vegetables, because Vitamin A increases resistance to tissue penetration by parasite larvae.

GUIDELINES FOR PARASITE CONTROL

- Filter all drinking water regardless of the source, or drink distilled water. Do not purchase any water

185

filtering system without making sure it removes microscopic parasites.

- Wash all foods thoroughly. It is optional to bathe them in ½ teaspoon Clorox to one gallon water for ten minutes, or one ounce of three percent hydrogen peroxide to one pint of water for ten minutes, and rinse well (especially chicken, fish, and meat). All fruits and vegetables should be rinsed several times after washing. If eggs are soiled, wash well and dry before breaking them open.

- Eat out as little as possible; food handling is a good source of parasites in most restaurants. If your lifestyle requires you to eat out often, or you just enjoy eating out, it is more important than ever to do a colon cleanse two or three times a year.

- Deworm your animals twice a year. Even indoor animals get worms.

- Make sure children who play outside, or anyone gardening, wash their hands, and scrub under their fingernails before eating.

- Wear gloves when cleaning up animal or human waste, or at least wash your hands *thoroughly*.

****Periodic detoxification and cleansing is a must for optimum health. You are NEVER completely free of parasites. **Always** do a colon cleanse at least two to three times a year!!! **THIS IS MAJOR HEALTH PROTECTION FOR EVERY PART OF YOUR BODY!**

[] [] [] [] [] []

DETOXIFICATION becomes important when you believe that **TOXIFICATION** is a reality. **TOXIFICATION** refers to the accumulation of toxic wastes in the cells of the body so that normal function is distorted or prevented. **TOXIFICATION** refers to the accumulation of toxic wastes from inadequate nutrients to nourish organs and tissues. **WHEN TOXIFICATION EXISTS ... YOU BECOME ILL!!!**

THE FOLLOWING ARE WAYS YOU ACCUMULATE TOXINS:

1. **EXTERNAL TOXINS** are various non-food substances taken into the body like the chemicals in food, water, air, and synthetics. A newspaper article written 20 years ago said we had formulated our 200,000th chemical. That seemed like a lot then, but nothing compared to the millions formulated today.

   "PROGRESS" MEANS NEW CHEMICALS ARE BEING FORMULATED ALL THE TIME FOR THE "NEW AND IMPROVED" OBSESSION WE HAVE IN THIS COUNTRY.

   The body is capable of making most normal chemical exposures inert, storing them in the body, or excreting them through the elimination systems. *THIS TAKES ENERGY "BORROWED" FROM NORMAL BODY FUNCTION, AND ALLOWS LESS NUTRIENTS AND BODY ENERGY FOR THE ACTIVITIES THAT **KEEP YOU HEALTHY**. Electromagnetic polluted frequencies also rob your body of the energy needed for normal body function. All this adds up to internal toxicity!*

2. **COMBINED CHEMICALS** IN THE SYSTEM MAY BE MORE DANGEROUS THAN ANY OF THEM SINGULARLY. There are second and third generations of combined chemicals, for which there is virtually no research available on how they affect the body.

3. **BY-PRODUCTS OF METABOLISM ACCUMULATE WITHIN THE CELLS BECAUSE OF POOR INTRACELLULAR ENERGY AND DEHYDRATION. THIS CAUSES CONGESTION, LIKE FIVE O'CLOCK RUSH HOUR.**

ATP (adenosine triphosphate) is the source of energy for the cell. ATP activates your sodium and potassium pump that is the "electrical" energy of your cell. Potassium is high on the inside of a cell, and low on the outside. Sodium is low on the inside of a cell, and high on the outside. Minerals have a magnetic pull from high to low, so potassium is always trying to get out, and sodium is always trying to get in. The sodium-potassium pump keeps these minerals in balance in the cell by "jerking" potassium in if it goes out, and "jerking" sodium out if it goes in. This jerking action produces the electrical energy of your cells in the same way a temporary magnetic field changing direction from North pole to South pole, induces an electromagnetic field (EMF), producing electrical energy. Without electrical energy activating intracellular chemical reactions, your cells would not be able to utilize nutrients correctly. Anyone with low energy, chronic or acute health problems, overweight or underweight, has one degree or another of low intracellular energy.

4. **WASTE PRODUCTS ACCUMULATE THAT SHOULD BE ELIMINATED BY THE EXCRETORY ORGANS.** This causes a toxic overload on the system, like two lanes of traffic being directed to one lane. The whole body is interrelated, and all systems need to help each other for best body function. *ANYTHING* you can do to protect the excretory organs is actually detoxifying the body. If one area is unhealthy, it puts a tremendous strain on the other areas.

READ ON TO LEARN MORE ABOUT THOSE WONDERFUL EXCRETORY ORGANS THAT PROTECT YOUR HEALTH ...

LUNGS:

Lungs depend upon proper breathing to take in oxygen, which is the first requirement of life. A deep inhalation floods your 750 million air sacs with new oxygen. Deep exhaling eliminates toxic gases filtered from the blood passing through the lungs. BREATH IS LIFE! When you forget how to breathe, you start dying. You must understand the importance of fresh air and correct breathing. Breathe from the diaphragm, *NOT THE UPPER LUNGS*, to get the full benefit of the body's assistance with air exchange. You should take at least three deep breaths, multiple times daily. You may need to find ways to remind you to deep breath until it becomes part of your day. Consider deep breathing when you get out of bed, before you go to bed, at every red light when driving, during television commercials, when you are fixing meals, or any other reminder. JUST DO IT!!!

If you have chronic respiratory symptoms you need to check out allergies as a possible cause. Work on all the "laws" of wellness to improve the health of the lungs. To protect the respiratory system DRINK YOUR WATER; AND ELIMINATE OR REDUCE MUCUS-FORMING MILK, DAIRY PRODUCTS, BEEF, and other mucus forming foods.

If you live in a new home or trailer, work in a new office, live or work with a smoker, or live in environmental air pollution consider antioxidants like A, C, E, zinc, selenium, grape seed, lipoic acid, or green tea extract.

You need to eat a diet that does not feed and encourage overgrowth of Candida yeast and parasites, as both organisms favor the lungs, and can be very destructive to the lung cells. *ANOTHER VERY GOOD REASON TO DO A COLON CLEANSE TWO OR THREE TIMES A YEAR!*

189

*Our medical profession is dealing with epidemic levels of sinus and respiratory crisis situations. While each is treated as an acute problem, no one addresses the real culprit ... **stressed out immune system**. The first place to start in protecting your immune system is to understand all the ways that can compromise it.* Look at the following list and see how many relate to you:

- EATING REFINED AND PROCESSED FOOD
- POOR DIGESTION AND ABSORPTION
- NUTRITIONAL DEFICIENCIES
- FOOD ALLERGIES
- pH IMBALANCE – TOO ACID OR TOO ALKALINE
- CONSTIPATION OR DIARRHEA
- INTESTINAL PARASITES
- OVERGROWTH OF YEAST AND FUNGUS
- INSUFFICIENT EXERCISE, LOW OXYGEN
- CHEMICALS IN FOOD
- ENVIRONMENTAL CHEMICALS
- CONTAMINATED WATER
- POLLUTED ELECTROMAGNETIC FIELDS PRODUCING POLLUTED ENVIRONMENTAL FREQUENCIES
- TOO MANY POSITIVE AND NOT ENOUGH NEGATIVE IONS IN THE ENVIRONMENT
- STRESS FROM POLLEN, MOLD, AND DUST ALLERGIES
- ALLERGIC REACTIONS TO BED MITES
- SOCIAL DRUGS, PRESCRIPTION DRUGS
- SMOKING, OR BEING AROUND SMOKERS
- EXCESSIVE CAFFEINE OR ALCOHOL
- SURGERY, ACCIDENTS AND INJURIES
- BACTERIA FROM ROOT CANALS
- MERCURY VAPORS FROM OLD DENTAL FILLINGS
- LOW SELF-ESTEEM AND LOW SELF-WORTH
- NEGATIVE THINKING AND LOW MOTIVATION
- POOR STRESS MANAGEMENT

By now you are stressed out just reading the list. All these sources of stress are discussed in this book, so relax and enjoy your learning journey. *Learning self-responsibility in health care should be only temporary stress, while lack of knowledge can plague you with a lifetime of chronic or acute illness! Consider yourself in school for the most important degree of your life!*

KIDNEYS:

The kidneys need your maximum amount of water daily to do their job. Increase your normal amount of water by two glasses in any acute inflammatory condition, or during a colon cleanse. **DO NOT LET YOURSELF GET THIRSTY!** Thirst can also be a sign of both *under-hydration* or *over-hydration*, so calculate your daily intake carefully!

The kidneys filter over 4000 quarts of blood daily. *The kidneys have three functions:*

* Prevents dehydration, and maintains normal water balance. Over-hydration or dehydration puts a tremendous strain on the kidneys.

* Forms urine, to throw off waste products.

* Keeps the body from becoming too acid or too alkaline.

Some people absorb water differently, and because of hereditary factors will become easily OVERHYDRATED. If you are overweight and have overweight relatives, you should evaluate whether you are a **HYDRIPHERIC TYPE**. This is discussed in *THE CHEMISTRY OF MAN* by Bernard Jensen. *Evaluate the following, and if you say a **strong yes** to more than half of the list, consider the program recommendations following this list:*

191

- *Emotions are calm, easy-going, gentle, and compassionate.*

- *Odors are easily detected, critical judge of food. Highly developed sense of touch, hearing, and smell.*

- *Diet preferences include soup, juicy dishes, and liquids.*

- *Imaginative and suffers in secret. A hydripheric type does not show emotions, fantasizes, has few friends besides close family, is subject to jealousy and may never get over love disappointments.*

- *Concerned with trivial happenings rather than major events. Disappointments cannot be forgotten or forgiven.*

- *Systems waterlogged and weakened causing poor digestion and absorption of nutrients. Illnesses are exhaustive.*

- *Metabolism is abnormal due to excessive tissue moisture; brain is sluggish.*

- *Appears healthy and robust but is actually ill and lacking vitality; resistive and recuperative powers are low.*

- *Joints and muscles are structurally weak.*

- *Reproductive system is weak; menses heavy or irregular.*

- *Susceptible to heat and light; easily chilled.*

- *Soft, delicate skin that is predisposed to skin and scalp diseases.*

- *Gain weight if you drink water based on one ounce for every two pounds of body weight.*

192

RECOMMENDED PROGRAM FOR
HYDRIPHERIC TYPES

- **Consume a high vegetable diet except starchy vegetables.** One problem in obesity is too much starch in the diet. In Hydripheric types, starchy vegetables (beans, peas, soy, peanut, potato, sweet potato, buckwheat, and squashes), and grains make changes in the digestive process that turns almost all food into **sugar.**

- **Eat foods high in organic sodium, and the trace mineral chlorine,** that help reduce cellular water. *If you are correctly hydrated, have a normal pH, and rotate all organic fruit, vegetables, nuts, seeds, and proteins, you will get organic sodium and chlorine from your diet.* Use solar or sun evaporated seasalt, or Celtic salt. Remember, organic sodium buffered in the whole salt complex, is a natural food that should be healthy in moderation. This is not the same thing as refined salt!

- **Consume <u>no more</u> than eight glasses per day** *total fluid* **intake** including soup, cold or hot drinks, rice or soy milk. Add *one* extra glass for inflammation or cleansing, *one or two* for severe obesity.

- **Eat protein foods in moderation.** Red meat is not recommended due to generally poor digestion.

- **Obtain** *essential fatty acids* in whole grains (in moderation), cold-pressed oils, nut and seeds (in moderation); or take supplements like Flaxseed, Black Currant Seed, Borage oil, or Emu oil.

- **Take short showers;** no long baths, saunas, whirlpools or swimming.

193

-   **Do bouncing-type exercise daily** (a minimum of 15 minutes), because Hydripheric types have lymphatic obesity discussed in the Internal Energy chapter.

-   **Consider that some people may do better in a dry climate.**

Correct hydration is a critical issue in weight control. There is a flood of information available on weight loss, but in my opinion it can be misleading, incorrect, or incomplete. Weight gain or problems controlling weight are complex issues, and should be handled from all aspects of physical, emotional, mental, and spiritual. Addictive patterns need to be understood. "Dieting" can cause more problems than it helps. When you attempt to diet, your body's metabolic rate slows down so that you store more of the food you are eating as fat, than you would if you were not dieting. When you go off the diet, you quickly accumulate more fat, because your body is programmed to think another "famine" could strike at any time.

Once you are drinking your correct amount of water, it is recommended you consider a colon cleanse. Know if your oral temperature is 98.4 to 98.6 degrees, before you judge the success or failure of any weight loss program. *Your goal should be "health," and not just weight loss.*

The following are guidelines for weight control:

1. Eat three sensible meals a day following the principles in this book. NEVER SKIP A MEAL! If snacks are needed between meals, eat only raw vegetables.

2. It is disastrous for weight control to eat a heavy meal before going to bed. Never eat after 8 PM!

3. Drink eight glasses (or one ounce for every two pounds of body weight if you are not a Hydripheric type) of

filtered water daily. Do not drink city water, or unfiltered well water. You may add lemon for taste, or just add it because lemon is an excellent food for the liver.

4. Losing weight is partly a question of increasing the efficiency of the digestive organs. Overweight or underweight is at least partly due to insufficient enzymes to correctly transform and utilize food. This can go back to low thyroid *activity* from either thyroid or adrenal stress. It is very important to include essential fatty acids like Flaxseed oil, Hemp oil, Black Current Seed oil, or Emu oil in the daily routine. Essential fatty acids activate the glands to produce enzymes needed in a healthy digestive process. *BUT FIRST, YOU MUST BE CORRECTLY HYDRATED, AND HAVE A BALANCED pH.* If your pH is not normal, consider taking a plant digestive enzyme supplement with meals. Be careful the enzymes are not from beef, or in a beef gelatin capsule.

5. Low body heat prevents nutrients from being burned for fuel and energy, and instead stores them as fat; or they are lost as toxic wastes. You should check your temperature monthly. For an oral temperature less than 98.4 degrees, follow the information in the thyroid section of the Internal Energy chapter.

6. Exercise is vital, because aerobic or oxygen-using capacity causes a subsequent increase in your metabolic rate (how fast you can burn calories). Deep breathing, taking three deep breaths at least three times daily is very important. Exercise is by far the most effective method of burning excess fat. *Exercise, visualize and grow thin!*

7. Losing weight too fast makes it harder to keep weight off because you also lose muscle. Chromium Picolinate increases muscle mass so that you burn more fat, and

prevents yo-yo dieting. Because muscle weighs more than fat, at first you may gain weight, and lose inches, before you lose weight.

SKIN:

The skin is the hardest working organ of elimination in the body. It frequently struggles against ...

- synthetic clothing that does not breathe. Recommend that clothing be cotton, wool, silk, or vicose rayon (some inexpensive rayons are synthetic). You may have a few select special clothing items that are synthetic, but you should make an effort to reduce your synthetic wardrobe. Your liver has to work harder when you wear chemical clothing. Natural is not just better in food ... it is better in clothing as well!

- invisible layers of toxins that are not removed by daily skin brushing.

Body brushing ...

- removes dead layers of skin and impurities.
- opens, and assists in cleaning the pores.
- revitalizes and increases eliminative capacity of skin.
- stimulates glands.
- stimulates nerve endings.
- contributes to healthy muscle tone and fat distribution.
- rejuvenates the complexion.
- improves general health that slows down aging.
- reduces microscopic mites in your bedding.

- lack of perspiration due to insufficient exercise.

- chlorine in city water; concentrated in bathing, long showers, and swimming. Chlorine is very drying to the skin. You are breathing in chlorine gas in your warm, steamy bathroom if you are using unfiltered city water. At least keep the bathroom door partly open to let the stream escape.

- a coating of cremes that clog cells rather than healing from the inside out. Many commercial products contain the wrong kind of alcohols, waxes, and rancid animal products that produce drying, and promote inflammatory problems. In our society of so many toxic and chemical based cosmetics, skin and hair products, I cannot say enough good things about companies that have made a serious effort to improve these valuable supporting health aids. *Commercial skin care products are often based on profit interests, instead of health concerns. You may pay a big health price for the superficial pleasures of some chemical and animal based skin care products.* **Skin health is an important part of body health. You absorb 60% of what goes on you skin, so evaluate skin care choices carefully!**

- poor nutrition, digestion, and elimination; and not enough **water**.

- free radicals created by the sun's ultraviolet radiation penetrates the skin, and damages the cells. You should wear a sunscreen even in the winter.

The top of your skin is made up of a tough material that forms a barrier against life-threatening organisms. While it is protecting you, it is disappearing right before your eyes. The entire population of cells in your skin is replaced once a month. To conserve heat, the skin constricts blood vessels, raises body hair and the skin around the hair causing "goose bumps." To cool you, the skin dilates blood vessels and activates the sweat glands which lowers temperatures on the skin, and the blood near the surface. This cooled blood flows back into the system, and cools other areas of the body. *Your skin works hard for you, and deserves a chemical and animal free cosmetic line,*

197

your correct amount of water daily, exercise to clean the pores, a good daily brushing, chlorine-free bathing, and natural fiber clothing.

LIVER: (Digestion chapter)

BOWEL:

The bowel is your sewage system of your body. By abuse and neglect, the bowel can become dangerously foul!!! This contributes to an overgrowth of microorganisms that stresses digestion, and contributes to an unhealthy liver.

OTHER SECRETIONS OF LESSER IMPORTANCE BUT STILL PART OF ELIMINATION are secretions from eyes, ears, nose, throat, and emotions of anger, joy, and sorrow.

ACCUMULATION OF TOXINS IN ALL THESE AREAS PRODUCE A SIMILAR RESULT ... DISTORTED, DELAYED OR PREVENTED CELLULAR ACTIONS, THAT ARE NECESSARY FOR THE PREVENTION OF DISEASE, AND FOR THE PROTECTION OF LIFE.

[] [] [] [] [] []

YOU, THE UNIQUE INDIVIDUAL

The way a person handles emotional or mental stress, the amount of exercise, and whether thoughts are coming from positive or negative energy, are all important factors in how each person deals with the PHYSICAL STRESS of *ACCUMULATED* TOXINS. Each person's body reacts uniquely to *toxic stress*, so one person with toxicity may develop arthritis, another cancer, and another maintain a surprising level of health.

Periodically the body tries to cleanse itself by various "acute" conditions like the common cold or flu. Remember, a cold means you are *struggling* with the build up of toxic waste. The flu means you are *losing the battle* against the build up of toxic waste. Stress is very important, and can put the system already toxic into rebellion. Only those with a "ripe" toxin accumulation that needs eliminated, and the immune system is suppressed, will develop a cold, flu, or infection.

LEARN TO TUNE INTO BODY LANGUAGE. A COLD IS NOT BAD LUCK. IT IS YOUR BODY TELLING YOU THAT YOU ARE TOXIC, AND YOUR IMMUNE SYSTEM IS DOWN!!! A COLD, FLU, OR INFECTION SHOULD BE TELLING YOU *LOUD AND CLEAR* THAT THE MENTAL, EMOTIONAL, AND PHYSICAL LIFESTYLE YOU ARE LEADING IS NOT WORKING. THOSE INCONVIENENT ILLNESSES ARE TELLING YOU *LOUD AND CLEAR* THAT YOU NEED TO EVALUATE HOW YOU ARE LIVING YOUR LIFE!!! DO NOT WAIT UNTIL DISEASE WRECKS YOUR LIFE. YOUR BODY TALKS TO YOU WITH MANY NAGGING SYMPTOMS. A SYMPTOM IS BODY INFORMATION THAT YOU ARE NOT WORKING AT A HIGH LEVEL OF FUNCTION. LISTEN TO YOUR BODY WHEN A SYMPTOM FIRST STARTS ... OR A DISEASE WILL MAKE YOU LISTEN LATER!!!

[] [] [] [] [] []

THE MAJOR CAUSE OF TOXEMIA IS CONSTIPATION...THE BIG C!

Even *before* the health of this country got so out of hand, Harvey Kellogg, M.D. of Battle Creek, Michigan (sound familiar?) performed over 20,000 operations, and found less than 10 percent of the patients had healthy colons.

THE CHOICE IS YOURS NOW! YOU CAN PAY THE HIGH COST FOR THE TREATMENT OF DISEASE, OR ASSIST YOUR BODY IN MAINTAINING HEALTH BY EATING AND DIGESTING HEALTHIER FOOD, AND INCREASING ELIMINATIONS NATURALLY.

199

Nature is the only one who cures. The best we can do is to help, and not hinder. We can immobilize the fracture with a cast, but it is not the cast that heals the fracture; the body heals itself. We should learn not to use modern medicine's arsenal unless it is an emergency. Once stable, go back to fundamentals so you cure the root of the problem ... not just knock off one of the branches.

[] [] [] [] [] []

THE INTESTINE IS OFTEN A MAJOR AREA FOR THE BEGINNING OF DISEASE. WE SADLY KNOW MORE ABOUT TUNING OUR CARS THAN WE DO ABOUT OUR BODIES.

Many people struggle with health problems without realizing the "cause" that can start in the bowel. **Leaky Gut or Leaky Bowel Syndrome** is something some people have heard about, but too few fully understand. We struggle with chronic poor health, allow symptoms to be treated instead of looking for the causes.

The lining of the gut is permeable, so small particles of food are able to pass through into other cells of the body. In a healthy body, the larger molecules and toxins from which the body needs protection, are kept contained by this lining. In Leaky Gut, the lining becomes porous and irritated.

All food substances pass through the liver before entering our circulatory system to be carried to other tissues and organs. The liver of people with Leaky Gut works overtime to remove oversized food molecules, and neutralize gut toxins, that consume antioxidants in large quantities. This miracle of detoxification of chemicals, and elimination of digestive wastes by the liver comes at a high cost.

The intestinal barrier is damaged from poor digestion, dehydration, viral and bacterial infections, Candida yeast, parasites, possible drug damage, and too little oxygen. In "Leaky Gut Syndrome" the gates of the gut are open too

200

wide and set the stage for inflammatory and infectious bowel diseases, inflammatory joint and muscle pain, skin conditions, food allergic reactions, pancreatic insufficiency, cancer, chemical sensitivities, hyperactivity, chronic fatigue, and liver dysfunction. Increased gut permeability may play a primary role in causing disease, or may be a consequence of it. By causing immune system reaction, liver dysfunction and pancreatic insufficiency, it creates a vicious cycle. The original cause may never be known, but once the condition has developed it can be self-perpetuating.

Your practitioner can measure your gut permeability through the lactulose/mannitol challenge test. A physician can call client services at the Great Smoky Diagnostic Laboratory at 800-522-4762, and get information on ordering the urine kit. The sugars are ordered separately either from that lab or a pharmacy.

With just a suspicion of the problem because of symptoms, even without formal testing, much can be done to improve your health in many ways. The lining of the intestine has the fastest production of new cells of any tissue in the body. A new lining is generated every three to six days. That is why it is important that the nutritional demands of this rapid cell turnover be met, if a damaged gut lining is to heal. Consider the following:

1. **Metabolism** is of prime importance since a nutrient-dense diet is necessary to turn around a leaky gut. Refer to the thyroid section in the Internal Energy chapter if your oral temperatures are less than 98.4.

2. **pH** must be balanced.

3. **Trace minerals** are important to improve cellular activity. Diet alone may not provide what is needed if you are dehydrated, and have poor digestion.

4. **Essential fatty acids** in whole grains, cold-pressed oils, nuts and seeds, ground flaxseeds, or

201

supplements like Flaxseed oil, Hemp oil, Black Current oil, Borage oil, or Emu oil aid digestion.

5. **Bowel flora** *products supply good bacteria.*

6. **Colon cleansing** *gets rid of parasite eggs, Candida spores, heavy metals and toxic wastes deeply hidden in pockets and folds, that are not always removed by daily elimination.*

7. **Liver herbs** *like licorice, milk thistle and dandelion support this overworked system. Foods good for the liver are* **lemon, beets, and olive oil***.*

8. **Amino acid products** *like soy protein, Lewis Laboratories Brewers Yeast, spirulina and blue-green algae, help in the regeneration of gut cells.*

9. **Diet** *should be milk-free, dairy-free, and red meat-free. Include fresh vegetables, and all the principles of the parasite diet to control Candida yeast and parasites.*

10. **Avoid unnecessary drugs** *that damage the gut.*

11. **Avoid alcohol** *that enlarges gut pores.*

12. **Avoid toxic chemicals, and food additives** *that the liver must handle.*

13. **Hydration** *is necessary to release hydrochloric acid into the stomach. This controls unhealthy gut bacterial overgrowth. Unwanted bacteria can destroy the protective mucous coating of the gut. People struggling with bowel problems may not be getting the full value from their filtered water. Consider water that has been energized, and is not*

dead water. One testimonial is my 11 year old cat's
bowels improved dramatically on energized water.

14. **Chew your food thoroughly** *to improve digestion, and*
    increase salivary epidermal growth factor, that
    stimulates tissue repair.

15. *Amino Acid Glutamine is a key factor in digestive tract*
    health.

Your efforts need to be concentrated for at least three
months, and maintenance should be a version of what helped you
heal.

[] [] [] [] []

Africans, with their high-fiber vegetable diet and large, wet,
unformed stools have little hospital huts. Many constipated
Americans, with their red meat, white bread, and small tubular
stools, have multi-story hospitals. **Most people living in
modern society today are constipated with one or both of the
following types:**

-   *One type is present when the feces that pass from the*
    body are overly packed together.

-   *Another type is present when old, hardened feces*
    stick to the colon walls, and do not pass out with
    regular movements.

Both types are so common in our society that scarcely
anybody recognizes them as being unnatural. Many people
consider *ANY* daily, or every other day movement (regardless of
the amount, or time of day) as normal. Few people have any
idea how much old, hardened bowel material is present in their
bodies. After a colon cleanse, one of my clients stated she
passed a piece of metal she swallowed 20 years before.

POSSIBLE PROBLEMS FROM WASTE PRODUCT
ACCUMULATION IN THE COLON:

- **ALTERNATING DIARRHEA AND CONSTIPATION,** because our American diet is like glue. Mucus-forming substances adhere to the intestinal walls, and as each layer develops, the tissues become thickly covered and less functional. Diarrhea can simply be a bad condition where the intestine is so badly clogged that the solids are held back; with only a small hole open, just the liquids are getting thorough. Anytime you have diarrhea you could lose valuable cell salts, and this loss could prevent diarrhea from improving. Replacing these cell salts (available in health food stores) could play a valuable role in assisting the body to improve symptoms for both human and animal diarrhea.

   The "virus bug" and bad food get blamed for a lot of diarrhea! Abdominal pain and cramps often clear up after the laxative and enema preparations needed for X-ray exams. If the doctor finds nothing wrong, he or she may order unnecessary drugs to relieve symptoms. Symptomatic treatment is a poor substitute for finding the CAUSE of constipation and/or diarrhea.

- **LOW BACK PAIN** may be caused by toxic poisons retained in the bowel, irritating the nerves.

- **HEADACHES** that are not explained by dehydration, food allergies, chemical sensitivities, Candida yeast, or parasites may improve as the system is detoxified.

- **FATIGUE** can result from general toxic build-up.

- **REDUCED LEVELS OF THE B VITAMINS** produced in the colon. The loss of these nutrients can contribute to many symptoms in our stress oriented world.

- **INTERFERENCE WITH THE ABSORPTION OF NUTRIENTS** into the bloodstream.

- **IRRITATED NERVE ENDINGS** that can lead to spastic or inflammatory conditions anywhere in the body.

- **TOXIC POISONS WHICH DETERIORATE THE WHOLE BODY** can contribute to cellular malfunction.

- **BLOODSTREAM GETS THICK WITH MUCUS** (undigested protein), so the waste from cells cannot be removed properly. This can lead to chronic inflammatory conditions.

- **BODY MUST CARRY AROUND EXTRA WEIGHT** that could be up to 10 pounds. Unless otherwise indicated, any weight program should start with a colon cleanse first.

- **INTESTINAL MUSCLE ACTION (called peristalsis) BECOMES SLUGGISH,** and fecal material backs up. Since moisture is re-absorbed, a hard stool is formed, and can contribute to hemorrhoids. If you have hemorrhoids, you may be low in Bioflavonoids, a part of the Vitamin C complex that assists in small blood vessel strength.

- **EXPOSURE TO INCREASED LEVELS OF ESTROGEN** because excess circulating estrogen is not broken down by the liver, and excreted in the bile or urine. *In chronic constipation, re-absorbed toxins put such a load on the liver, it cannot properly break down excess circulating estrogen. Added to the "look-alike" estrogen from agriculture chemicals, the overload can create many health problems. Practically every person on the planet is being exposed to certain environmental pollutants, synthetic chemicals, and detergents that "mimic" the effects of estrogen in the body. Correcting constipation is critical in preventing epidemic numbers of breast cancer, or other estrogen-dependent cancers, or non-cancerous tumors.*

Adding the other "laws" of wellness can greatly improve your risk factor.

SIX REQUIREMENTS FOR HEALTHY ELIMINATION:

1. **Water -** Your correct amount of distilled or filtered water daily!!! For most people this is *at least* eight glasses of water daily. You should increase your water by one to two glasses a day if you have an infection, or bowel elimination is hard, or you have done strenuous exercise.

2. **Fiber** – With enough fiber , your movement will be …

   - **large amount** (a comfortable feeling you have eliminated enough). Multiple "urgings" throughout the day with minimum elimination is not normal.

   - **soft, wet and bulky** (more like formed cow droppings, or soft tubular). If movement is packed tubular, YOU ARE CONSTIPATED!

   - **low in odor** (some people will have more odor based on diet and herbs).

   - **passed quickly** without straining (no magazine racks needed) one time *BEFORE* noon; even better, another later in the day.

KINDS OF DIETARY FIBER (some foods contain both):

   - **INSOLUBLE FIBER** does not dissolve; it provides bulk and helps in the movement of food and water through your intestine.

- **SOLUBLE FIBER** dissolves: it lowers cholesterol, detoxifies bile acids, controls appetite, and slows absorption of glucose.

VALUES OF DIETARY FIBER:

- **Holds water and provides bulk** that moves food quickly through the digestive tract. Water and bulk combine to make fiber an effective cleanser, moving through your intestines like a sponge picking up wastes, toxic debris and pollutants along the way. The bulkier, softer stool means less strain and pressure on your bowels, and their blood vessels.

- **Reduces toxic waste**, since food that is held up in the small intestine too long (due to lack of water and fiber), causes fermentation and putrefaction to occur. That toxic waste floods the bloodstream and produces internal toxemia and disease. *YOUR COLON IS NOT A STAINLESS STEEL HOLDING TANK! THE COLON CAN HOLD EIGHT OR MORE MEALS WORTH OF UNDIGESTED FOOD AND WASTE, WHEN CONSUMING THE TYPICAL WESTERN DIET. WITH AN ADEQUATE FIBER DIET, ENOUGH WATER, AND EXERCISE, THE COLON HOLDS ABOUT THREE MEALS.*

- **Decreases re-absorption of bile salts** that are meant to be eliminated. This creates a *need* for the liver's cholesterol stores to make more bile acid, and that lowers blood cholesterol levels. Bile acid normalizes intestinal flora, and decreases growth of unhealthy micro-organisms.

- **Speeds elimination, and decreases calories absorbed**. Excess fat and sugar is excreted, instead of raising triglyceride levels, stressing the pancreas, or causing weight gain.

3. **Exercise** - gets nutrients to the cells, and removes toxic waste at a speed that allows the body to work at optimal performance or heal itself. Exercise also encourages the progressive wave of contraction in the bowel, called peristalsis.

4. **Balanced pH of the body.** Discussed in the Digestion chapter.

5. **Control of Candida yeast and parasites.** It is very important to practice the "parasite" diet guidelines on a daily basis in your home, as a lifetime commitment to wellness. On social and special occasions, you may tolerate a favorite treat. If you start to have chronic symptoms, you may be *socializing* too much!

6. **Healthy stress management.** People want health to be as easy as getting rid of a headache with an over-the-counter drug. Your results may be disappointing if you only work on the physical symptoms, and not deal with the spiritual, mental, and emotional needs. Decide on a goal, build your future, put value in your life, improve your self-esteem, and understand your basic needs. This will help balance pH, and improve a lot more than elimination. Read Chapter 1 again!

[] [] [] [] [] []

RECOMMENDATIONS TO IMPROVE ELIMINATION

A BALANCED pH IS A PRIMARY GOAL. If your pH is not normal you must make that **top priority.** Read the Digestion chapter again. *All recommendations will be temporarily successful if you do not follow the six requirements for healthy elimination just discussed.*

The following recommendations are based on general health of the elimination system. **If for any reason your medical** history includes current problems in the stomach, intestines, liver or gallbladder, you should *contact your medical doctor and have a complete evaluation.* *If all tests are normal but you still have symptoms, then you may want to consider one of the following:*

-   **Herbal elimination formulas** are not like "laxatives" that only force elimination. Herbal formulas help heal the body because they also support the health of interrelated systems. If ingredients like psyllium seed constipate you, it is most likely due to *not enough water.* As your elimination becomes healthier, you may be able to reduce your intake of elimination supplements. *BE MORE CONCERNED ABOUT CONSTIPATION THAN DEPENDENCE ON NATURAL HERBAL PRODUCTS THAT STIMULATE THE WHOLE DIGESTIVE SYSTEM.*

-   **Natrum Muriaticum Cell Salts** may help to balance the fluid in the intestines, if the movement is hard or loose.

-   **Fenugreek** is an intestinal lubricant and can be healing for sores, ulcers, and other irritations in the intestines. Two delicious drinks are:

    (1) 1/2 teaspoon fenugreek, 1/2 teaspoon mint, 1/2 teaspoon comfrey, and two star anise in a cup of hot water, with honey optional.

    (2) Check you local health food store for herbal laxative teas.

-   **Natural fiber products like seaweeds** are very helpful in colon health.

-   **A high fiber diet** means foods in their most natural form.

    Unrefined foods include ...

- brown rice and whole grains, instead of refined or processed.

- fresh fruit with skin and seeds if edible, instead of drinking juice. Kiwi, berries, bananas, pears, apricots, peaches, cherries, pineapple, figs, and apples are high fiber fruits.

- whole grain cereals and breads contain high fiber and bran. Toast bran with sesame or sunflower seeds for casseroles or dessert toppings.

- nuts or seeds for snacks, or chopped in recipes or salads. Add flaxseeds and psyllium seeds to soups, stews, and casseroles.

- unpeeled potato, sweet potato, and vegetables. All vegetables contain fiber, especially dark green, leafy ones. Make sure you scrub non-organic potatoes well, and cut out all the "eyes." Potatoes can be sprayed with a fungicide, mold retardant and sprout inhibitor ... it is best to buy organic.

- beans; precook and freeze for quick meals. Make bean soups and freeze for future meals. I have a "soup day" when I stay home and make two different recipes that give me several months of quick frozen meal choices. All dried and fresh beans (legumes) are high in fiber.

- seaweeds that contain trace elements often missing in today's food, and contain bulk cellulose for your high fiber diet. Check Oriental markets and health food stores for many different varieties.

* *There is no fiber in meat, fowl, fish, seafood, dairy, eggs, fats or oils.*

- **Grapes** are excellent to secrete bile that stimulates the intestines. Eat whole grapes with skin and seeds. Grape juice may be high in mold content, and is high in simple carbohydrates. Grapes can be heavily sprayed, so purchase organic.

- **Drink regularly throughout the day, and do not get thirsty.** You should drink ½ to one glass of water 15-30 minutes before meals, and the rest spread out over the day for best hydration. *Forgetting to drink, and then drinking large amounts to catch up, will only flush out nutrients, enzymes, hydrochloric acid, cell salts, and make you urinate more frequently.*

- **All fresh fruits and vegetables** are good for the intestines. Carrots help to liquefy bile, which is your body's natural laxative. Cooked fruits and vegetables cause great loss in potassium needed for intestinal movement, call peristalsis. If the liquid left after cooking vegetables is a small amount, drink it, or freeze and save for soups. Do not discard those valuable minerals! Diets high in refined salt can cause low potassium levels that will interfere with good elimination. *This is no time for the typical American fast food, and overcooked diet.*

- **Blackstrap molasses** is a natural laxative, and a source of iron and calcium; it is a simple sugar, so use in *moderation*. As a hot drink, put one teaspoon or more in hot water.

- **Prunes** create waste-washing action from their rich potassium. Prunes are simple carbohydrates, so consume in *moderation*. Pour one cup of boiling water over a few prunes, cool, and consume before breakfast. You may not tolerate dried fruit if you are mold sensitive, or have Candida yeast overgrowth symptoms. Heated food high in mold will lose the reproductive properties of the mold, but not the allergic response.

211

- **Garlic** has a laxative effect and is rich in potassium. GARLIC IS ONE OF YOUR BEST FOOD FRIENDS. Garlic dissolves wastes and propels them toward elimination channels; a powerful blood cleanser. One clove a day, or deodorized garlic supplements, helps keep your bloodstream clean. Many people have an unknown milk and beef allergy. Garlic may come in a beef capsule, so like all supplements, you should start looking for your choice in a vegicap, caplet, liquid, softgel, or tablet.

  Garlic has cleansing elements that have a beneficial effect on the entire system. Garlic stimulates the appetite and secretion of gastric juices, promotes peristalsis in the intestines, eliminates intestinal parasites, aids the elimination of poisons from the body through the skin pores, is antibacterial and antiviral, and has a cleansing action on the kidneys. **WHAT A FOOD!!!**

- **Aloe Vera juice** with its superior nutritive and cleansing qualities is excellent for intestinal problems. Months of Aloe use may be needed to turn around chronic colon conditions. The *quality* of Aloe varies **greatly.** Some Aloes are very refined and have little therapeutic value, so do not settle for less than unrefined, whole leaf, cold-pressed, and concentrated Aloe.

  Aloe Vera has been well documented, and worthy of consideration for the following uses:

  - A natural cleanser.
  - May relieve pain associated with joints and sore muscles.
  - A helpful addition to bacterial, viral, and fungal control.
  - Dilates capillaries, increasing blood supply in the area to which it is applied locally.
  - May reduce the fever or heat of sores.
  - Anti-inflammatory.
  - May be helpful in itching symptoms.

212

- Nutritional, as it provides a wide range of nutrients, including mucopolysaccharides for healthy joints.
- Digests dead tissue including pus through the action of enzymes, hastening healing.
- Moisturizes the tissue.
- Safe to use for animals with similar problems.
- An FDA approved safe food. It has been taken internally by all ages from infant to elderly throughout the world since 400 years before Christ.

- **Olive oil** is an excellent natural laxative. It stimulates the liver, and gallbladder, and lubricates the intestines without blocking absorption. Consider taking one teaspoon two times a day, in rice or soy milk; or use in cooking *daily.*

- **A relaxing defecation schedule**. Do not set the morning alarm so late that you have to rush. If you know you cannot have an elimination until you eat breakfast, then eat when you first get up, and not just before leaving the house. Because of the circadian rhythm cycle for elimination ending at 12 noon, you can create body imbalances having your main elimination later in the day. *Some people will not eliminate until the next day if they miss that cycle.*

- **Tranquility in eating**. Remember digestive and elimination systems are interrelated, and both are greatly affected by emotions.

- **Exercise** mechanically stimulates the intestines. A stooped or relaxed posture induces constipation by weakening the abdominal muscles. An erect posture exercises the muscles of the trunk, encourages correct breathing, and healthy blood circulation. If your circulation becomes sluggish, there can be a toxic buildup in your cells. Discomfort may be due to an injury or infection, but INTERNAL TOXEMIA can show itself as PAIN.

[] [] [] [] [] []

THE INTERNAL HOUSECLEANING

A good housecleaning really helps after six months of surface dusting and vacuuming. *Your intestines and entire body need extra attention twice a year also, to get rid of hidden build up of toxins, and waste products.* If this sounds scary or unappealing, listen to all the options and I am sure you will find one choice that is acceptable. You DO have choices ... reduce the chances of getting sick and aging too fast ... or dying too soon.

Some people cannot fast without food while they are cleansing because they are hypoglycemic or diabetic, underweight, too ill, too active, or need a certain level of energy for a demanding lifestyle or job. Cleansing is still possible with normal modified meals. If you are concerned about cleansing based on your medical history, you should *first check with your doctor.*

ALL CLEANSING RECOMMENDATIONS SHOULD START OUT ON A LOW DOSE, AND WORK UP TO SUGGESTED DOSE AS TOLERATED!! There is a safe cleanse for everyone. ***BEFORE CONSIDERING ANY CLEANSE YOU MUST BE DRINKING YOUR ·REQUIRED LEVEL OF WATER, EXERCISING TO MOVE THE LYMPHATIC SYSTEM, AND DEEP BREATHING EVERYDAY!*** The lymphatic system is discussed in detail in the Internal Energy chapter. **YOU CANNOT CLEANSE IF YOUR BODY IS NOT FLOWING!**

CLEANSING OPTIONS TO CONSIDER WITH MUCUSLESS MEALS

CHOICE #1:

Consider a modified mucusless diet outlined in Dr. Christopher's *3 DAY CLEANSE, MUCUSLESS DIET* (refer to Resource References). The mucusless diet followed for one month ... or a lifetime, will provide a gentle cleansing.

214

The body loves it! *For the purpose of cleansing, the mucusless diet has some changes:*

- Eliminate all commercial refined and processed foods.

- Eliminate refined sugar and commercial sodium chloride salt.

- Eliminate eggs (or only use occasionally in recipes).

- Eliminate red meat (beef, pork, lamb, buffalo, deer, and elk).

- Substitute soy, rice, oat, coconut, or nuts for any milk need.

- Eliminate all refined flour products. Consume only 100 percent whole grain products which are mucus forming when cooked, but allowed because of their nutritional value and fiber.

- May have hormone and antibiotic-free chicken or turkey, rabbit, emu or ostrich, fish; seafood only socially because they are bottom feeders picking up waste and toxic matter. Allowed are fresh fruits, raw vegetables, cold-pressed oils, raw nuts and seeds, and natural sugars.

CHOICE #2:

Consider a good colon cleansing product available in health food stores. If you are elderly, weakened by chronic illness, or have chronic bowel problems, you may want to try the first cleanse by cutting the directions in half. If tolerated, you may decide to try the full recommendation for the next cleanse. Follow the mucusless diet in Choice #1 for one month ... or a lifetime.

CHOICE #3:

Take *unrefined* Aloe Vera juice starting with one teaspoon one time a day for two days, then two teaspoons for two days, then one tablespoon for two days, then one and 1/2 tablespoons for two days, then two tablespoons (one ounce) daily for two or more bottles. Increasing the dose depends on the degree of symptoms, and your state of health. Some people tolerate two tablespoons at one time. Others do better taking one tablespoon in the morning, and one tablespoon at night. Aloe Vera is an excellent general cellular cleanser, and assists in repairing the digestive and elimination systems if the Aloe is concentrated therapeutic quality. Follow the mucusless diet for two months ... or a lifetime.

CHOICE #4:

The amazing fruit of *Tahitian Noni* has been used by the Polynesians for over 2,000 years for a wide range of health related conditions. This is not a testimonial for Noni, but you might consider the option after reviewing the published information. XERONINE in Noni is reported to be involved in numerous cellular reactions that are believed to control cellular regeneration and aging. Cell aging leads to the breakdown of cell and organ function, which causes disease formation in the body. Taken internally XERONINE may work at the molecular level to repair those damaged cells. Noni can be applied locally to open wounds, abrasions, cuts, or burns, and may accelerate the healing process. Noni is reported to enzymatically accelerate the removal of dead tissue, increases oxygenation, and stimulates immune response. Start with one teaspoon daily for two days, then two teaspoons for two days, then one tablespoon for two days, then one and ½ tablespoons for two days, then two tablespoons (one ounce) daily. Like Aloe, Noni may be better tolerated taking one tablespoon in the morning, and one tablespoon at night; available in health food stores. Follow the mucusless diet for two months ... or a lifetime.

CHOICE #5:

Consider the benefit from cleansing with Flor-Essence (either liquid, or make your own tea at home). The same product under a different name is called Essiac. Most health food stores will carry one or the other. Recommend you follow bottle instructions, but start slower with one teaspoon one time a day, and work up to maximum dose. Your cleansing symptoms will be a lot worse if you are not hydrated and exercising. Flor-Essence or Essiac have been mentioned for chelating out mercury toxicity from old mercury fillings, and needs to be considered for at least three months. Cilantro (available in tincture form in health food stores) is an herb helpful in chelating out mercury. Follow the mucusless diet for two months ... or a lifetime.

CHOICE #6:

Take the lemon juice cleanse as described in CHOICE #2 in the next section dealing with fasting cleansing options. This cleanse can be done non-fasting, and follow the mucusless diet for two months ... or a lifetime.

CHOICE #7:

Dandelion, red raspberry leaves, and thyme are good cleansing teas to add to any cleanse choice. An excellent "Spring Tonic" tea is Elder Flower, known for its ability to clean out the wastes that accumulate in your bloodstream. Follow the mucusless diet for two months ... or a lifetime.

MY PERSONAL YEAR AROUND CLEANSING PROGRAM INCLUDES A COLON CLEANSE TWO TIMES A YEAR, AND ROTATE MANY BODY CLEANSING PRODUCTS. CHECK YOUR HEALTH FOOD STORE , OR MY WEBSITE FOR UPDATED RECOMMENDATIONS. THIS IS A LIFETIME COMMITMENT. YOU OWE IT TO YOURSELF TO PROTECT

YOUR HEALTH BY ATTEMPTING TO KEEP TOXIC WASTES ON THE MOVE!!!

[] [] [] [] [] []

BODY CLEANSES THAT REQUIRE FASTING

Fasting without food may not be tolerated by everyone. Some people need food to take certain medications. **Never stop any medication for any recommendation in this book without clearing it with your doctor.** Some people with low blood sugar or diabetes, on multiple prescription drugs, or demanding physical jobs will do better on one of the cleanses that allow you to eat a mucusless diet. *For those who choose to cleanse while fasting, consider the following choices:*

CHOICE #1:

Dr. Christopher's *3 DAY CLEANSE, MUCUSLESS DIET* as discussed in the book.

CHOICE #2:

Lemon juice cleanse for one, two, or three days depending on your state of health, activity, work, and dedication as follows:

1. Before the fast I recommend a *pre-cleanse* routine to prepare the body for easier cellular cleansing. If the bowels have not been moving before noon daily, you should consider an herbal laxative formula for two weeks. During this time, hydrate your body with your correct amount of water, exercise, and deep breathing daily; and follow the mucusless diet.

2. When you are ready to do the cleanse, add the juice of six to ten fresh lemons to two quarts of distilled or

filtered water; lightly sweetened with maple syrup or raw honey optional.

3. Drink only the two quarts of lemon water, plus any distilled or filtered water you need for your body weight over the two quarts. You may dilute the lemons a little more by adding extra water, instead of adding as much sweetener. Drink all of the two quarts of lemon water each day. Consume two cups every three hours, alternating with more plain filtered or distilled water as allowed for your weight.

4. If necessary, you may munch on any raw vegetable.

5. Each day consume from 1/4 to two teaspoons of olive oil three times a day. If tolerated, increase to one tablespoon three times a day to cleanse the gallbladder and liver. *START OUT WITH A LOW AMOUNT TO TEST YOUR TOLERANCE.* Too rapid cleansing with olive oil can cause nausea, and/or pain on the right side. If symptoms occur, stop the cleanse until symptoms subside. **For severe symptoms, contact your doctor. Cleansing the gallbladder can loosen stones, and if one causes a blockage it can be serious. Do not hesitate to go the emergency room for unreasonable distress!**

6. After three days of tolerated cleansing, on Day Four, return food slowly to the system. Add fresh vegetables and fresh fruit first.

7. Day Five, add white chicken meat, or vegetable protein.

8. Day Six, add other mucusless foods; *continue* mucusless diet for one to two months ... or a lifetime.

CHOICE #3:

Fasting should always be done with filtered or distilled water to rid the body of toxic wastes. Fasting one day a week on either plain water, water with fresh lemon juice; fresh organic apple, or organic grape juice, could add health filled years to the average American. Do not fast on liquids alone for more than four days. Any day you fast, include olive oil, so the gallbladder is also cleansed. Follow a liquid cleanse with a mucusless diet for two months ... or a lifetime.

[] [] [] [] [] []

THINGS TO REMEMBER IN CLEANSING

- Discontinue all supplements during a **fasting** cleanse, but *continue taking prescription drugs.* If medication needs to be taken with food, you should pick a non-fasting cleanse.

- If cleansing produces a cold, flu-like symptoms, or an increase in old symptoms, that is a sign of the **real need for cleansing**, as your body moves toxins out of the system. If you are too symptomatic, stop the cleanse. Follow a mucusless diet for one month with your correct amount of water, walk 15 minutes 3 x a day until better, and deep breath *daily*; and then try cleansing again.

- If you do not have a bowel movement every day on a cleanse, take an herbal laxative as needed. *DO NOT CONTINUE TAKING CLEANSING RECOMMENDATIONS IF YOU ARE CONSTIPATED, NOT DRINKING YOUR CORRECT AMOUNT OF DISTILLED OR FILTERED WATER DAILY, AND EXERCISING TO MOVE THE LYMPHATIC SYSTEM.* If constipation or diarrhea is experienced, you will need to judge what program you are on, to determine if changes must be made.

- You could feel weak on a cleanse as your body works hard internally. Use this time to rest and catch up on reading, TV, and hand work.

- Start it when you have several days off to evaluate reactions. It is important to do at least 15 minutes daily of lymphatic exercise options *during a cleanse*, but no other strenuous choices, or exercise longer than 15 minutes *at one time.* During any cleanse, your body is *working hard inside.* Cleansing can be a miracle for the body, but if you do not follow the recommendations, you could have unnecessary discomfort.

- You did not become toxic in a few days, so be patient and realize it may take multiple cleanses to regain your health. You will find a favorite cleanse, and you should do it two times a year for *Spring and Fall housecleaning. It is a lot easier to prevent the build-up of toxic wastes then to cleanse a toxic body!!!* In this stressful world it would be wise to consider one of the many choices listed ... and consider eating a mucusless diet most of the time.

- To help *remember to drink* while on a liquid cleanse, set a kitchen timer.

- There may be weight loss due to the body discarding waste. These are all signs of building health. In health, weight will normalize. If weight *loss* would be a problem, you should pick a cleanse that allows you to eat a mucusless diet, rather than a **fasting** cleanse.

- You must *first* deal with an existing medical problem, and alter your cleanse to fit your needs. A person with Candida yeast symptoms, allergies, diabetes, heart disease, or being treated for any disease, must first think of those limitations before selecting a cleanse or modifications. *REMEMBER: ANY VERSION OF ANY CLEANSE, OR ANY LENGTH OF TIME IS BETTER THAN NO CLEANSE AT ALL. A*

221

MUCUSLESS DIET ALONE IS A CLEANSE. **If you have any concerns due to your past medical history, first check with your attending physician.**

[] [] [] [] [] []

For far too many people the health of the intestines is in crisis. With all the antibiotics we have taken in the last 80 years both in our food and from medication, our good intestinal flora is seriously out of balance. Without intestinal flora, we can eat and still be malnourished. Antibiotics kill the friendly bacteria as well as the bad bacteria. Imbalances produced by this abuse has set us on a collision course with germs … and the germs are way ahead. Rare diseases considered to be illnesses of the past are now emerging worldwide.

"Life-saving antibiotics are losing their effectiveness and eventually will cure as well as a sugar pill."

- World Health Organization,
Press Release, September 27, 2000

The more we go about killing germs, the more we weaken our resistance. When we abandon what is natural we start hosting degenerative diseases. In desperation we accept heroic measures that gamble with life. A place to start is refusing to eat animal products containing hormones or antibiotics. You should be very cautious about taking antibiotics for physical symptoms unless a culture proves it is not viral, and other options cannot be safely considered. BE CONCERNED THAT VIRUSES OR BACTERIA ARE UP BECAUSE YOUR IMMUNE SYSTEM IS DOWN! Living by the "laws" of wellness will make you less likely to be faced with an acute crisis. If you must take an antibiotic, you should consider taking a milk free acidophilus product twice a day on an empty stomach, at double the recommended dose for two to three months. Before you exhaust yourself in discouraging chronic symptom chasing, EVALUATE

YOUR IMMUNE SYSTEM!!! Preventive medicine in this area could be life saving!

[] [] [] [] [] []

DETOXIFICATION IS CELLULAR ASSISTANCE FOR A LONGER LIFE!!! **ONE OF THE BEST WAYS TO DETOXIFY YOUR BODY IS TO ADD OXYGEN!!!**

*Too many people breathe shallow breaths, and do not exercise enough to encourage deep breathing. The earth's oxygen supply is rapidly being reduced with rampant deforestation. Add to that overeating, nutritional deficiencies, chemicals in our food and water, and you have a body starved for oxygen. The results of "oxygen depletion" are fatigue, depression, loss of concentration, poor judgment, irritability and a long list of chronic and acute health problems. People die in their own waste. You can put a sack over your head and be dead very quickly. **THE ONLY WAY YOU ARE GOING TO LIVE A HEALTHY LIFE IS TO ROUTINELY REMOVE THOSE TOXIC WASTES FROM YOUR BODY!!!***

WE LIVE OR DIE ON A CELLULAR LEVEL. The cleaner your bloodstream and your lymphatic system, the healthier your body. Every part of your body is washed, nourished, and oxygenated by your bloodstream every second of your life. Without a supply of clean, oxygenated blood, your tissues and cells will age ... and degenerate.

The substance that removes waste in the planet is ozone. Oxygen is a two molecule atom, and ozone is a three molecule atom. The third molecule combines with a pollutant, and oxidizes it, which converts the pollutant to another form that is not damaging. The ozone level is considered a level of pollution, but it really is the planet's ability, or lack of it, to protect itself from the build-up of pollution. High ozone levels also mean high pollution. Ozone is a very powerful oxidizer. As

223

early as World War I it was used in the treatment of wounds. It has become an alternative to chlorination, being used in the largest ozone water purification center in the world in Los Angeles.

The same process happens in your body when ozone is applied to a virus, bacteria, fungus or plant physiology ... it oxidizes it, and destroys it. If you had enough oxygen in your body, it would produce the ozone needed, because the electrical charges in your body actually produce ozone. Ozone acts as a beneficial scavenger, efficiently destroying diseased cells and invading organisms through the oxidation process.

An example of slow oxidation is rust, and fast oxidation is fire. In the body some types of oxidation are harmful, and produce free radicals. Your best protection against the damage of "negative" oxidation is to take antioxidants like Vitamin A, E, C, zinc, selenium, grape seed, lipoic acid, and green tea extract. Other antioxidants are in herbal formulas. We know there would be no life if certain oxidation did not occur. The body uses oxidation as its first line of defense against bacteria, virus, yeast, and parasites. Without oxidation we die very quickly.

One good way to supply extra oxygen is hydrogen or magnesium peroxide ingestion. Everyone knows about hydrogen peroxide for first aide, Few people know how powerfully it can heal if taken in a more concentrated form. Health food stores carry hydrogen peroxide products, and the books that will educate you on the value of oxygen products. Many supplement companies are now producing oxygen products with enthusiastic information and testimonials. *NEVER TAKE AN OXYGENATING PRODUCT WITHOUT ANTIOXIDANTS!* Hydrogen peroxide is not a cure-all, but incredible successes have been well documented in dozens of conditions. It is up to the individual to investigate all opportunities to encourage body healing in a way that "first does no harm." That is what self-responsibility in health care is all about.

Healthy cells love oxygen, and there are some natural ways to add oxygen. You can inhale therapeutic quality essential oils like frankincense, sandalwood, myrrh and clove. Any chlorophyll-rich food like green vegetables, spirulina, and blue-green algae oxygenates the blood. Therapeutic oxygen spas are becoming the health spas of the future. For more information check the website www.oxytherapy.com.

[] [] [] [] [] []

We have covered Positive Thinking, Nutrition, Digestion, and Elimination. Self-responsibility in health care would not be complete without knowledge of general exercise. Even more important, the **right kind of exercise for the lymphatic system.** When you add all these basic subjects to understanding body hydration, pH balance, Candida yeast and parasite control, digestion, absorption and utilization of nutrients, you are now capable of treating the CAUSE of disease and not just the symptoms.

You are getting close to the end of your beginners course on wellness, so to complete your power to heal, read on ...

CHAPTER 5

INTERNAL ENERGY

If I told you all you needed for good health was a daily banana split, you'd probably rush to the nearest ice cream store…and you would *LOVE* my book! We would all like health to be easy … and fun. If you are like many people, you may believe that is not possible. Well, you are wrong. Health *can* be easy … and fun!!!

Many school age children love Physical Education class. They do not realize that their happy positive attitude and deep breathing is good for their health. Too often, those playful children mature into serious, goal-oriented adults. If we lose our youthful enthusiasm for life, it can become very difficult to establish exercise habits just for enjoyment. The exercise we do establish is often associated with social or business opportunities.

At about age 40, or sooner, our bodies begin to slow down. Unfortunately, just about the time you realize you have lost a degree of health, you may be too sick, too tired, or too overextended in your lifestyle to make healthy choices. **If you are not in any acute state of poor health, you may decide to put things off until tomorrow … or, think bad problems happen to the other guy.** When problems do happen, you may be too willing to let a medical professional keep you going with a "quick fix." IF YOU DID LOSE CONTROL OF YOUR HEALTH … IT IS SIMPLY A MATTER OF CHOICE TO GET CONTROL BACK! Following the laws of wellness, drinking your correct amount of water, and exercising *daily* is the place to start.

It is not important what you play … it is just important that you play. Play may be the most vital thing you do! FITNESS is the key word to enjoying life to the fullest, on all levels of spiritual, mental, emotional, and physical. There are many books available that recommend exercise to overcome the tendency towards overweight, poor circulation, constipation, and

226

multiple diseases. THIS CAN HARDLY BE CONSIDERED FUN!!! FITNESS SHOULD BE A LOT MORE THAN PREVENTING DISEASE ... IT SHOULD ALSO BE ENJOYABLE!!!

[] [] [] [] [] []

WHAT MAKES ONE PERSON EXERCISE, AND ANOTHER SHOW NO INTEREST?

Your decision to exercise is based on more than your physical condition. It is your state of TOTAL WELLNESS ... like getting up in the morning and looking forward to the day. You may not have any physical symptoms, but you may still be unmotivated; if you have emotional or mental symptoms YOU JUST DO NOT CARE TO EXERCISE! Negative emotions or negative thinking can interfere with your *enthusiasm*, even if you are free of physical symptoms. Acute problems are generally on the physical level, but most other times, symptoms are mental or emotional as well as physical. Learn how all these levels influence your life, and it will help you understand why you make certain choices.

MENTAL PROBLEMS are thinking problems. Thought processes can have a powerful influence on our motivations. A positive thought might be, "I think it is a great idea to go." A negative thought might be, "I don't think I'm up to going." Negative mental thinking can inhibit your ENTHUSIASM.

There is a difference between poor mental health and poor mental attitude. You may need medical supervision for mental illness, but you can decide through WILL AND DETERMINATION to improve your ATTITUDE. Remember to say your positive affirmations. It will always be easier to consider fitness when you are coming from POSITIVE ENERGY.

With dehydration, the level of energy in the brain is decreased, and many symptoms like fear, anxiety, insecurity, emotional problems, and depression can become a major

227

deterrent to healthy choices. A depressive state caused by dehydration can lead to chronic fatigue ... and that can greatly affect the desire to exercise.

***EMOTIONAL PROBLEMS** are feeling problems. Unfulfilled basic emotional needs lead to frustrations that can affect enthusiasm. POSITIVE EMOTIONS lead to happiness and the desire for social contact, motivation and physical activity. NEGATIVE EMOTIONS lead to unhappiness and withdrawal. You might cancel an intended walk after a disagreement with a friend ... and none of the excellent books on exercise will make a difference in your decision. If you are emotionally upset, you are very likely to decide not to walk at all.*

***PHYSICAL PROBLEMS** in our society have become the comfort zone for excuses. Emotional and mental states are generally not necessary to mention, because giving an excuse that you have a headache is so socially accepted. You are much more likely to say to someone you do not want to be with, "I'm too tired," rather than, "I'm upset with you." THIS EASY PHYSICAL EXCUSE MIGHT BE USED ANYTIME YOU DO NOT WANT TO DEAL WITH A PROBLEM.*

[] [] [] [] [] []

HOW DO YOU DEVELOP ENTHUSIASM TO BE A PARTICIPANT IN LIFE?

1. Start every day with **POSITIVE THOUGHTS AND AFFIRMATIONS.** When you open your eyes in the morning, think about the miracle of being alive. *THIS IS YOUR DAY! WHAT ARE YOU GOING TO DO WITH IT?*

2. Everyday, **BE WILLING TO BE FLEXIBLE.** When petty irritations get you down, allow yourself the luxury of only a short negative period. Since nothing can be done in a

negative state, the sooner you think more positively, the sooner you can get on with life. It is your *CHOICE* how you interpret your daily events.

3. Everyday, attempt to **DISCOVER WHY YOU DO NOT FEEL WELL,** instead of suppressing and masking *chronic* symptoms with drugs, that do not treat the cause. There is a need for medical professionals to work together. In an acute crisis, modern medicine's approach is comforting, and can be life saving. After the crisis, we must always look for the *CAUSE* that made the body not work at optimum performance.

4. Everyday, **BE OPEN TO NATURAL TREATMENTS** that *improve* your constitution ... *YOUR VITAL ENERGY FORCE!*

> *If you have a symptom, your vital force is down! It is your depressed vital force, not your symptom, that is the origin of disease. To change your level of health you must change your constitution or "VITAL FORCE," a subtle governing energy that organizes and directs physical and chemical action in the body. Efficiency of your vital force is reflected in degrees of health ... or illness.*
>
> *Symptoms are an expression of your vital force's effort to heal. Do not suppress your body's attempt to communicate with you!!! Learn to tune into body language!!! Drugs that suppress chronic symptoms should be avoided if possible.* **I am not referring to drugs used in acute or emergency situations, or drugs used for management of body systems like thyroid or diabetes.** *Just treating chronic symptoms is* **masking** *the fact that your vital force is down. You need to deal with that, rather than just temporarily wanting to feel better.*

229

FACTORS THAT INDIRECTLY AFFECT VITAL FORCE

- **Therapy or medication for mental symptoms:**

   A natural way to treat mental and emotional symptoms is with Bach Flower Remedies. They are in the same category as other subtle methods of healing. They are available in health food stores in tincture form, or from some holistic practitioners in homeopathic form. The Bach Flower remedy system heals by restoring harmony in awareness; they act more on the energy system rather than the physical body.
   The healing energies are released from the flowers in a way that there can be no overdose, no side effects, and no incompatibility with any other treatment. To use flower remedies requires no training, but only the ability to acknowledge your thoughts and feelings. There is no true healing unless there is a change in outlook, peace of mind, and inner happiness.

   IF THIS DOES NOT SOUND PROBABLE, THEN UNDERSTAND BACH FLOWER REMEDIES HEAL IN A WAY THAT "FIRST DOES NO HARM." POSITIVE AFFIRMATIONS ARE NEEDED TO REPROGRAM THE SUBCONSCIOUS.

   Simplicity has to do with unity, perfection and harmony. That is the reason everybody feels attracted to the "simple things in life." The further your research advances, the greater you will realize the back-to-basics simplicity of all creation. Refer to the Positive Thinking chapter for more insight into the different Bach Flower remedies.

- **Psychotherapy, counseling, or Bach Flower Remedies** for emotional symptoms.

230

- **Supplements; medication for acute symptoms; food, chemical, or environmental testing and treatment; chiropractic and other alternative health care programs** that improve body function; and other forms of therapy for physical symptoms.

One way to give your vital force a boost and improve your sense of well being is to increase physical and mental energy with negative ions. Ions are charged molecules of air. Over open land there are about equal numbers of negative and positive ions. When that balance is disturbed, there is trouble for all forms of life. Sprawling cities, automobiles, pollution, smoking, modern synthetic fibers, new building materials, chemical products, modern transportation, central heating and cooling systems in sealed office and apartment buildings, all are part of the man-made environment that has too few ions of both kinds for healthy, normal life.

Atmospheric ions can affect your health, well being, efficiency, emotions, and mental attitude. Negative ions are called "happy ions," and positive ions are "grouchy ions." More than half of the population of North America spends the majority of their time in cities and urban areas, where the total ion count is hopelessly depleted.

So, if you live and work in our "new and improved world," are tired, fight with the family, suffer from tension, anxiety, depression, have erratic days and listless nights with below par sexual interest, you may be suffering from an overdose of positive ions. Some people are far more sensitive than others.

The most noticeable beneficial effect of using negative ion generators is to repair the damage done by man himself to the air we breathe, and the world in which we live and work. Negative ions are unlikely to cure anyone of anything. Their most noticeable effect, however, is to give us more energy, both mental and physical, and improve our sense of well being. Check health food stores and health magazines for sources of negative ion generators.

231

FACTORS THAT DIRECTLY AFFECT VITAL FORCE

- **Acupuncture:**

   Acupuncture creates a smooth flow of vibratory energy throughout the body, by connecting with points on the pathways which relate to various organs, glands, and cells. Fine needles are inserted at certain points identified with body symptoms. By changing their distorted vibrational nature, balance is restored and the body can repair itself.

- **Spiritual healing:**

   Faith and hope have performed miracles for many who have a strong spiritual connection. To experience that connection, open up new strengths by uniting with your Creator. Do not underestimate the power of prayer. We frequently look for energy to survive our crisis oriented world, without making that learning experience easier by connecting to the peace within.

- **Homeopathy**:

   Homeopathy works on the principle of RESONANCE, like when a singer shatters glass on a special note that *matches* the energy of the glass. The source of a homeopathic remedy (like an herb) is "proven" to have certain symptoms when taken in excess. When these symptoms *match exactly* the symptoms of the person with a problem, the *two energies* when combined will increase the overall energy (called resonance). This increased energy raises your vital force and you are now stronger to overcome the symptoms. The importance in homeopathy is to match *alike symptoms* as much as possible on *all levels of mental, emotional, and physical.* The closer the match, the stronger the resonance. You will have no effect from the wrong remedy because there will be no resonance (like a singer who does not break glass).

I always carry an emergency kit of homeopathic and herbal ointments and formulas for sudden cold or flu symptoms, and injury or pain. Refer to Resource References for Homeopathic books and supplies. Understanding Homeopathy is a "first do no harm" approach to the management of chronic symptoms, as well as most non-life threatening acute symptoms. For all acute symptoms, first check with your doctor.

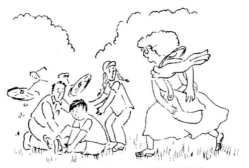

MOVE OVER! I'm an HERBALIST!

5. Everyday **THUMP YOUR THYMUS GLAND**. The word thymus is derived from the Greek work "thymos," which denotes life force. The thymus gland is weakened by six major factors: stress, emotional attitudes, physical environment, social environment, food, and posture. *To straighten the thymus gland:*

> *Place three fingertips into the indent of your neck, at the top of your breastbone. Slide fingers down on your breastbone one inch; tap the area with your fingers for about one minute, to energize your thymus. Repeat frequently for acute symptoms.*

233

6. Everyday be **FORGIVING OF YOURSELF AND OTHERS!** Destructive thoughts deplete your life energy ... *LOVING THOUGHTS INCREASE YOUR LIFE ENERGY!* Connect with your Spiritual force to help you find the peace within.

7. Everyday stand up straight. **THINK AND WALK WITH CONFIDENCE!** This is a positive energy factor. Good posture facilitates the energy flow through the body.

8. Everyday **REACH OUT TO SOMEONE.** Be willing to touch, show affection to someone, be caring and compassionate. Outstretched arms (as in reaching out) use both right and left brain for balance. Say *"I love you"* often to someone special.

9. Everyday put the kind of **MUSIC IN YOUR LIFE** that you enjoy. Music can give you pleasure, and that can encourage a sense of peace and calm. From that mental state you are more likely to accomplish something.

10. Everyday create **POSITIVE ENERGY**, because it can influence you, and those around you. *ENERGY IS CONTAGIOUS!* A weak person can make you weak (if that is your choice), and an energetic person in the room can energize you, *raising your life energy* (if that is your choice).

11. Everyday dress in a way that will **TURN *YOURSELF* ON!**

12. AND ... **EVERYDAY SMILE!** *LIFE IS WONDERFUL IF YOU "THINK" IT IS!!!* Your day may have a harsh challenge in it, but that should be an opportunity for learning, and a chance to become stronger.

    "I am healed when every cell in my body is smiling."

                                                    - Mary Eberdt

[] [] [] [] [] []

I HAVE A GOOD ATTITUDE, I'M READY ... WHERE DO I START?

Start by looking at exercise as a pleasant way to add relaxation to life's stressors, and pleasure to your day. The success of your exercise program does not depend on the exercise book you are reading ... but, on your *FRAME OF MIND*! Make a commitment to your future. Exercise is a private satisfaction. Exercise is something you do for **you**. If you do not give *"YOU"* a part of each day, look at what value you place on yourself. Are you coming from "I can't be happy, and life is hard?" Ballroom dancing is an exercise treat I give to myself. You should exercise for health's sake ... but also for pleasure. The two are self-supporting. The healthier you are, the more you will like to exercise, and the more you like to exercise, the healthier you will be.

[] [] [] [] [] []

FITNESS MYTHS:

Misconceptions keep people from becoming fit and healthy, such as:

- No pain, no gain.
- A person has to sweat to get in shape.
- Big muscles are important.
- Lots of protein makes a person strong.
- You must spend at least 10 hours a week in a fitness program to stay in shape.

KEY POINTS IN ACHIEVING FITNESS AND PROLONGING LIFE EXPECTANCY

- **LOWERING THE AT-REST HEART RATE:** That rate is determined by your level of activity maintained during the last four weeks. Simply by monitoring the heart beat, the level of effort and fitness can be determined at any point in time. The mortality rate for adults with resting pulse rates over 92, is four times greater than for those with pulse rates less than 67. You should take your resting pulse when you first wake up, **before you move.** Find your pulse on your wrist (the thumb side of your hand); or on your neck (down from your ear).

- **REGAIN FITNESS IN ONE MONTH**: 80% of an individual's fitness can be gained or lost in a 28 day period. A person who has not exercised in years, can regain fitness in one month by following some simple guidelines.

FIVE DAILY REQUIREMENTS FOR MAINTAINING FITNESS according to Lawrence Morehouse, director of the Human Performance Laboratory at U.C.L.A.:

1. Limbering includes two or three minutes of simple stretching, twisting, bending and turning.

2. Standing for a total of two hours during the day.

3. Lifting something heavy for at least three minutes.

4. Walking briskly for at least three minutes.

5. Any activity that will burn at least 300 calories a day. The list is long, but generally plan on something that keeps you moving at least 45 minutes.

236

IN ADDITION, SPREAD OUT THE FOLLOWING THREE TIMES DURING THE WEEK:

- One or two minutes of warm up; then five minutes of exercise that works the upper body, abdominal and legs.

- Five minutes of aerobic exercise that gets the pulse into the target range. This formula is for people who can safely increase their heart rate. Check with your doctor if you are not sure.

    Subtract your age in years from 220, and take 80 percent of that number to get your maximum heart rate. Healthier circulation will carry vital nutrients to all of your body structures, and eliminate toxic wastes. Do not exercise to exhaustion. In fatigue, you lose muscle strength three times faster than you build it. Regular exercise is safer because it builds stamina that protects you from sudden exertion. It is sudden exertion that can be damaging, or even fatal.

[] [] [] [] [] []

It can be a challenge to move if your back, neck, joints, and muscles hurt; some **ROOT CAUSES** are:

- *In the spinal column, water acts as a lubricant for contact surfaces, and supports 75 percent of the weight of the upper body. Once arthritis in any joint is established, it can be a lifetime sentence, unless the* **ROOT CAUSE** *is understood. Joint pain not associated with injury should be considered as* **local thirst**. *In a well-hydrated joint, friction damage to the cartilage is minimal.*

- *Another* **ROOT CAUSE** *of arthritis is from* **inorganic minerals**. *Your body cannot assimilate inorganic*

237

calcium and potassium minerals in well, spring, and city water. Most of these minerals pass out of the body, but some slough off into the joints and build up deposits; well, spring, mineral, or city water is not recommended. All water today should be filtered. Research and technology will replace energy lost in filtering water, and energized water is the water of the future.

- **Emotions** *can be a* **ROOT CAUSE** *of many physical symptoms. Holding resentments can be a factor in arthritis. Stress can be a factor in muscle pain and general fatigue. Read Chapter 1 again!*

- *An* **unhealthy diet** *must be a main consideration for* **ROOT CAUSES** *in any state of ill health. Read the Nutrition Chapter again! If you are not faithful to a healthy diet, you may not feel well enough to consider exercise options. Read the Digestion chapter again to improve your* **absorption** *of food. There is a real difference between eating the right food, and getting that nutrition into the cells. If nutrients are not correctly burned up for fuel and energy, they are lost as toxic waste, or stored as fat. Just feeling full, and not hungry, is not enough. We are a well fed society, and also a society full of chronic and acute illness.* **It is time people start thinking of food as "life giving", and not just for fun!**

[] [] [] [] []

IF YOU CAN BREATHE, YOU CAN EXERCISE!

Physical restrictions may limit your physical choices, but *mental and emotional attitudes may be far more inhibiting.* Start with DEEP BREATHING and POSITIVE AFFIRMATIONS.

To deep breathe, push your stomach muscles out; take in all the air you can. Let the air out slowly until you cannot let any more air out, and your stomach muscles are pulled in. The exhale should have a wheezing air sound coming from your diaphragm under your rib cage, not your throat. This is a full cleansing breath. BREATH IS LIFE! We learn to breathe at birth; when we forget how to breathe correctly, we start to die. Abnormal cells multiply in the absence of oxygen. Organic food and alive food supplements supplies the iron needed to carry oxygen.

[] [] [] [] [] []

WHY DO SO MANY PEOPLE STOP EXERCISING AFTER THAT FIRST BURST OF ENTHUSIASM?

Some people ...

- exercise out of fear of illness. They do not decide to exercise because they want to relax, and treat themselves to some pleasure. Fear is their motivation. Because *fear* is negative, it is likely they will have other negative attitudes, and find excuses not to continue.

- stop because they feel good, and would rather do something else. *They often take health for granted!!!*

- stop because the exercise was recommended treatment for a medical problem, which has been resolved.

- are pressured by others to join them, but low self-esteem and subconscious negative thoughts soon win over.

- like the choice of exercise to be more social; home equipment ceases to be fun in the garage.

- feel the choice is too strenuous for their endurance level.

239

- are unwilling to return to an exercise that resulted in an injury.

- feel the choice may be too time consuming for their lifestyle.

- feel the choice may be too stressful, or fearful ... like skiing.

- feel the choice may be too expensive to continue at this time.

- feel the choice may be too inconvenient because they have moved.

- feel the choice was not as much fun as they thought it would be. Be careful with this one. Are you coming from, "I can't be happy, and life is hard?"

BE WILLING TO STRETCH OUT OF YOUR COMFORT ZONE TO TRY NEW ACTIVITIES. TAKE A RISK ... BE ADVENTUROUS! ESTABLISH A PROGRAM TO FIT YOUR LIFESTYLE, AND THEN STICK TO IT UNTIL IT BECOMES HABIT!

[] [] [] [] [] []

EXERCISE OPTIONS HAVE IMPORTANT POINTS TO CONSIDER

SUPPLEMENTATION:

The supplements used for exercise of unusual duration and expended energy, need to be considered differently than daily maintenance with normal exercise. Your fitness trainer for endurance exercise should acquaint you with the adjustments needed in your nutrition program.

You may need a nutritional supplement that contains a natural sugar like fructose during heavy exercise. This will replace the sugar used in exercise, so energy is not pulled from the muscles, and cause fatigue. Sugar used at this time is replacement, and not the same problem as raising sugar levels when the body does not need more sugar. Parasites and Candida yeast feed off extra sugar in the diet.

THE FOLLOWING EXERCISE OPTIONS ARE GOOD FOR THE LYMPHATIC SYSTEM:

- **JOGGING**: If you are not a "conditioned jogger" it may *not* be the best recommendation to start. If you are not in good physical health, jogging can be very stressful to the hips, knees, and ankles on paved roads and sidewalks. Jog on an athletic track or sawdust trail, wearing the best running shoes. Jog with a friend or dog for safety. Long distance jogging is hard on the immune system.

- **STATIONARY JOGGING OR AEROBICS**: Purchase exercise tapes, follow television exercise shows, or join a health club.

- **TRAMPOLINE OR TREADMILL**: This is a safer form of jogging, easier on your joints, and more acceptable when time or weather is a problem. Recommend 15 minutes once or twice a day; becomes more social while watching television. If you are unable to jump due to physical limitations, you can still get benefit from a trampoline. Sit with your feet on the trampoline, and let someone else do the jumping. Small trampolines can be very inexpensive, but a more expensive one will have stronger springs to hold up under heavier weight. A trampoline or treadmill in every home makes 15 minutes of daily exercise easier, because it eliminates problems from a busy lifestyle, and the weather! YOU OWE YOURSELF 15 MINUTES A DAY, BECAUSE YOU ARE WORTH IT!!!

- **HIKING**: Getting back to nature is the best way to enjoy all the sensory groups … visual, auditory (hearing), kinesthetic (feeling), gustatory (taste with lunch or snack), and olfactory (smell).   This produces the best relaxation.   Joining organizations that enjoy the outdoors adds both friends and fun, such as Sierra Club, Audubon Society, or a photography club. THINK AHEAD … a little thought about food, water, clothing, shoes, bug protection, and emergency items are critical to the success of your adventures.

- **WALKING**: Shoes are most important; do not forget food, water, and clothing on longer walks. Walking is easier on the joints than jogging. Slow walking may be necessary at first, but fast walking is better for your lymphatic system. One way to indoor "walk" is with a treadmill, or march to music around the house.

- **ACTIVE BALL SPORTS**:   If your bones, nerves, and muscles are not healthy, you may be prone to accidents in contact sports.   If you have accidents due to constant *aggression* while playing ball sports, it may be an example of your frustration in life.

- **DANCING**: You do not have to go to a night club to dance. Turn the music on at home and put a little wiggle in your body. *LOOSEN UP … DANCING AROUND THE HOUSE WILL HAVE A WONDERFUL EFFECT ON YOUR LYMPHATIC SYSTEM, AND YOUR SELF IMAGE.* Smoke-free ballroom dancing is growing in popularity, because it provides wonderful exercise, pleasurable time with friends, is safe and friendly for singles, and great bonding for couples. *ANYTHING THAT PUTS PLEASURE IN YOUR LIFE PROMOTES HEALTH, BECAUSE YOU GET CIRCULATORY IMPROVEMENT FROM RELEASE OF TENSION. I HIGHLY RECOMMEND YOU TRY DANCING TO ADD HEALTH, AND PLEASURE TO YOUR LIFE.*

THE FOLLOWING EXERCISE OPTIONS ARE GOOD FOR CIRCULATION AND MUSCLE TONE:

- **BIKING**: Biking is fun; it boosts your circulatory system and reduces stress. *Always wear a helmet when biking,* because you have no control if a car hits you, or take a tumble from any number of other reasons. Today we jump in the car to go a block. *Choose to walk or bike short distances. Long distance biking can be hard on the immune system.* MODERATION IS A KEY WORD FOR HEALTH.

- **STATIONARY BICYCLE AND OTHER INDOOR EQUIPMENT**: Many people lose interest after the "new toy" period is over, especially if equipment is stored in an isolated area of the home. Exercise near a television, or join a health club.

- **SWIMMING**: This is particularly helpful if you have an injury or physical limitations. Swimming is less physically stressful to move under water. You can stimulate your whole body by applying pressure from the water jets to your hands and feet in a jacuzzi. All the meridians in your body terminate there. Do not stay in a hot jacuzzi more than 15 minutes; and only under the guidance of your doctor if you have high blood pressure.

- **YOGA, TAI-CHI OR OTHER STRETCHING CHOICES**: These exercises do not increase heart rate; they should be used in addition to active exercise choices. They are helpful to limber up the body, release tension, improve body alignment, improve circulation and energy flow, and to learn to appreciate body movements.

WE ARE ALL INDIVIDUALS. SOME ARE OLD AT 40, AND SOME ARE YOUNG AT 60. A LOT DEPENDS ON YOUR LIFETIME HABITS OF LIVING. IN PLANNING YOUR EXERCISE PROGRAM,

CONSIDER YOUR LIFESTYLE, BUT EVERYONE SHOULD HAVE AT LEAST A FEW MINUTES OF STRETCHING EXERCISES MORNING AND/OR EVENING. Do your routine the same time each day, as discipline is the key to your fitness program.

The prime essential in promoting any exercise program is good POSTURE. Poor posture can mean poor digestion, poor elimination, poor circulation, and set you up for fatigue that will sabotage your enjoyment of life. Be conscious of how you stand, sit, or work at a desk. To encourage good posture, stand with your back against the wall so your calves, buttocks, shoulders and back of head all touch the wall together. Raise both arms high overhead touching the wall ... lower arms, relax, and repeat five times each day.

- **SKIING**: The key word to remember is CLASSES. To prevent injuries, make sure you have some understanding of your general state of health, and have enough instruction to develop self-confidence. I did it wrong; injuries included a fractured rib, and the same year a broken hip. Try snowshoes if you would love to get in the snow, but downhill or cross-country is too frightening for you. If you can walk, you can snowshoe. The outdoor experience is worth it!!!

  If you exercise in the morning you will get almost 2/3 energy from stored fat and 1/3 from carbohydrates; in the afternoon, you will burn more carbohydrates. Burning fat is better for weight loss, so if you are overweight, exercise in the morning; exercise in the afternoon or evening if you are more concerned about general health than weight loss.

IN SUMMARY, HOW DO YOU DEFINE EXERCISE?

Exercise is an activity that *enriches* the life of a person who has mental, emotional, and physical energy enough to be enthusiastic about life. The decision to exercise is based on the decision to *enjoy life to the fullest.* The desire to *begin* exercise implies a degree of health in POSITIVE THINKING, NUTRITION, DIGESTION, AND ELIMINATION. The decision to *continue* exercise is a *definite* degree of health in POSITIVE THINKING, NUTRITION, DIGESTION, AND ELIMINATION.

[] [] [] [] [] []

STUDIES INDICATE THAT EXERCISE IS A DEFINITE FACTOR IN BLOOD VESSEL DISEASE

We have become oversensitive to the word "cholesterol." Your body needs cholesterol for vital body functions. The fact is, the less cholesterol you take in with your foods, the more the body makes; and the more cholesterol you take in with your food, the less your body produces. Either way the body will get what it needs. High cholesterol should tell you the body is struggling in some serious ways. Understanding the principles of hydration, elimination, and the health of the liver, is critical for anyone with high cholesterol levels. ALWAYS LOOK FOR THE **CAUSE** OF BODY STRESS!

Cholesterol production is a part of the cell survival system. Cholesterol makes the cell wall impervious to the passage of water, protecting cells against dehydration. Excess cholesterol production can mean cellular dehydration. After a period of a few months improving cellular hydration *ON A REGULAR BASIS, increased cholesterol production will be less required, and in time should decrease, unless there are other reasons.*

The restriction of cholesterol containing foods has very little to do with your cholesterol level alone. You must also consider body hydration, and health of the liver and elimination systems. People and doctors love tests! It is easy to measure blood cholesterol, and if elevated, is often blamed for atherosclerosis, when other causes are ignored.

245

THE ARTERIES' HEROES AND VILLAINS STORY

- *Cholesterol is manufactured in the body, mainly by the liver; it also goes to the liver from animal food you eat.*

- *In the liver cholesterol is loaded, along with triglycerides (a combination of fatty acids), into very-low density lipoproteins (VLDLs), which carry it through the bloodstream.*

- *After releasing their triglycerides into the body's tissues, VLDLs are transformed into different carriers, called low density lipoproteins (LDLs), which deliver cholesterol to the cells.*

- *Excess LDLs, rejected by the cells, help trigger the formation of plaque, which can build up in artery walls, and block free blood flow.*

- *The heroes, high-density lipoproteins (HDLs), work against this process by removing excess cholesterol from blood and cells.*

- *HDL may also be able to collect cholesterol from the plaque, reversing the process that leads to heart attacks.*

- *Once filled with excess cholesterol, the HDLs may deliver some of their cargo back to VLDL carriers, which then become LDL's as before.*

- *The liver removes LDLs from the bloodstream and converts cholesterol into bile acid, which is then eliminated through your daily bowel movement. If the bile acid is not eliminated because of **constipation**, cholesterol can recirculate back to the liver, and increase cholesterol levels.*

* *If total cholesterol is 160, ideal LDL is 100 or below.*

If total cholesterol is 200-240, LDL acceptable if 130 -160.
If total cholesterol is 240-300, high risk LDL is 160-200.
*If total cholesterol is above 300, there is an extreme high
risk if LDL if above 200.*

*It is recommended that your cholesterol and HDL ratio be
UNDER five. Ex: The HDL is 30 and the total cholesterol is
240, you have a ratio of eight, which is too high. If the HDL
is 80 and cholesterol 240, you have a low risk of three.*

Many people know what their cholesterol reading is because
they have had it checked fairly recently. But how many of you
are up on that other number on your blood-fat profile,
triglycerides? You need to check out the triglyceride story
carefully. This lipid (fat) could be more important to you than
the others.

The bad news is that if your triglyceride level is high (above
150), your risk of heart disease may be greater than if your
cholesterol is high. The existence of high triglycerides should
also serve as a red flag to look for conditions like Type II
diabetes, high blood pressure, and obesity. The good news is
that elevated triglycerides can be lowered promptly and
permanently without drugs. You need only to change your diet
to something that is not a textbook example of the "All-
American Buffet."

Evidence from the famous Helsinki heart study suggests that
high triglycerides are even more dangerous when combined with
low "good" HDL cholesterol reading. A triglyceride rise
indicates an excess amount of insulin, meaning this is purely a
carbohydrate disorder. A low-fat diet, in which you have no
choice but to eat more carbohydrates, can make a high
triglyceride level worse. *If your triglyceride test is high, I
suggest you follow these dietary guidelines both for prevention,
and normalizing abnormal readings:*

-   Swear off alcohol and simple sugars, meaning anything
    sweet, including fruit, fruit juices, milk and dairy
    products.

247

- Carbohydrates from starchy vegetables, grains, and tubers should constitute no more than 25 percent of your daily calories. Starchy vegetables are listed in the Nutrition chapter, but non-starchy vegetables are very low in carbohydrates, so you can have your fill. Retest triglycerides to monitor your progress.

NINE COMMON SENSE HEALTH CHOICES FOR CIRCULATION

MODERATION WILL ALWAYS BE THE BEST CHOICE IN THE SEARCH FOR HEALTH.

1. **BUTTER IS BETTER, AND ORGANIC BETTER BUTTER IS BETTER YET** (refer to Nutrition chapter). Butter contains important natural nutrients. For most people, cholesterol food eaten in *moderation* is not going to be the *main* villain in atherosclerosis.

2. **AN EGG IS A FOOD CAPABLE OF PRODUCING LIFE!** According to Dr. K. Donsbach, *"Eggs will not affect cholesterol or blood vessel disease state except to lower your cholesterol and make your body more disease resistant."* For most people eggs can be consumed in MODERATION! Eggs contain more natural lecithin than is needed to handle the cholesterol in the egg.

3. **CHEMICAL POISONS CAN CAUSE ARTERIAL IRRITATION.** *All the research on how chemicals affect our bodies may never be complete.* Do not purchase foods with added chemicals. This reduces the *overall load* on the liver, from the chemicals you *cannot eliminate* in the environment. Our society's obsession with new homes, new cars, synthetic materials, "new and improved" chemical *everything* puts a huge stress on

248

the body's ability to protect itself. *Antioxidant supplements listed are more important than ever before:*

- *Vitamin A captures free radicals which are unstable particles bent on damaging your cells. You need Vitamin A because of the world's upset balance of nature. You should not take more than 10,000 I.U. of Vitamin A daily, because excess can be damaging to the liver. Extra Vitamin A should be in the form of Beta-carotene, that can be stored in the skin, and changed into Vitamin A in the liver when needed. Vitamin A is needed to connect amino acids into a chain, to travel through the bloodstream. A high protein diet can deplete Vitamin A. This is not good in such a polluted environment.*

- *Vitamin E is the oxygen efficiency nutrient, and is concentrated in the pituitary, which is the master gland of the body. It is THE supplement to take if you want to reduce the speed of the aging process and protect life. My testing repeatedly shows you should use a **dry** rather than an oil E product.*

- *Vitamin C is the key nutrient used by your body to detoxify harmful substances, and help protect your liver. During stress, greater than normal amounts are lost in the urine. Vitamin C's co-factors (bioflavonoids) inhibit the destruction of Vitamin C by oxidation. Buffered Ester-C with Bioflavonoids may be better because our stressful society tends to be too acidic.*

- *Zinc deficiency greatly affects the immune system. Zinc is a powerful antioxidant, and has many functions in digestion, enzyme production, and cellular activity.*

249

- *Selenium* is deficient in most of our soil. It is very important in controlling chemical sensitivities. Brown rice has 15 times as much selenium as white rice. *THIS IS NO TIME FOR PROCESSED FOOD!!!*

- *Grape Seed Extract* is among nature's most potent antioxidant. Look for 100% proanthocyanidins in your supplement. Grape seed is the most powerful source of proanthocyanidins, and is a highly bioavailable complex that is rapidly absorbed.

- *Lipoic acid* is a universal antioxidant. It works throughout the body boosting glutathione levels in the cells, which is a protein that consists of powerful antioxidants. Lipoic acid helps eliminate toxic metals from the body, so it is helpful in mercury detoxification.

- *Green Tea Extract* is the most powerful antioxidant ever discovered. It is antifungal, antiparasitic, antibacterial, antiviral, immune stimulant, and cancer retardant. Available in both regular and decaffeinated tea, and concentrated vegicaps, it is a health treat for the body!

> "My research has proven that to live a long, healthy life you must control the free radicals unleashed in your body."
>
> - Dr. Earl Mindell

4. **DO NOT DRINK HOMOGENIZED MILK!** The process produces an enzyme called Xanthine Oxidase that irritates the lining of the circulatory system, and is highly suspected as a initiating factor in atherosclerosis. Goat's milk is naturally homogenized by nature, and raw milk is not homogenized. Using homogenized dairy

products in cooking is better for the circulatory system, because heat destroys Xanthine Oxidase. Soy milk and rice milk are both far more digestible, and less allergenic than cow's milk, and dairy products.

5. **THE BEST DIET IS ONE OF MODERATION AND COMMON SENSE.** Avoid commercially processed oils, refined flour and refined sugar in products. Steer clear of recommendations for "low this" and "high that" (which varies from book to book anyway). GET BACK TO BASICS!!! Do not overuse any one food.

6. **AVOID CONSTIPATION** to reduce the reabsorption of bile salts that were meant to be eliminated. This lessens the need for the liver's cholesterol stores to make more bile acid, and that can raise blood cholesterol levels. Never in the history of mankind has regular colon cleansing been more important because of modern day chemicals, diet, and stress.

7. **DRINK YOUR APPROPRIATE AMOUNT OF PURE WATER DAILY USING THE LATEST TECHNOLOGY.** DEHYDRATION IN THE CELLS ENCOURAGES CHOLESTEROL PRODUCTION TO KEEP FLUID IN THE CELLS.

8. **EXERCISE IS CERTAINLY NOT LAST WHEN IT COMES TO IMPORTANCE.** The benefits of a regular fitness program fall easily into three categories:

weight control - feeling of well-being - longevity

[] [] [] [] [] []

WHEN YOU EXERCISE YOU HAD BETTER KNOW HOW TO ABSORB CALCIUM

You may learn about CALCIUM the hard way, after you break a bone. Many people concerned about calcium levels obediently take a calcium supplement ... assuming that it is being absorbed. THIS IS AN ASSUMPTION YOU CANNOT AFFORD TO MAKE, BECAUSE CALCIUM IS THE MOST DIFFICULT OF ALL THE MINERALS TO ASSIMILATE!

Calcium is in every cell of the body. About 99 percent of body calcium is contained in bones and teeth. The kidneys produce a compound, and along with a hormone from the parathyroid gland, regulate the release and absorption of one percent that circulates in body fluids. Blood calcium levels do not tell the whole story! A blood test does not evaluate bone loss...only a bone density test will do that. Calcium moves in and out of the bones with about 600-700 milligrams being exchanged each day.

From birth to about age 35 we build bone; after that we gradually lose more than is being replaced, about three to eight percent each decade. Sun exposure, good nutrition, normal progesterone levels in women, and exercise can prevent or slow this process.

ROLES OF CALCIUM:

- Essential for healthy teeth.
- Helps to maintain the acid/alkaline pH balance of the body.
- Helps the blood to clot.
- Transports impulses along the nerves.
- Necessary for good muscle contraction.
- Important in brain functioning.
- Regulates the rhythm of the heartbeat.
- Initiation in some hormone secretions.
- Activation of enzyme reactions.

SOME SYMPTOMS OF LOW CALCIUM ARE:

- Inability to deal with stress. Calcium taken at bedtime can be a tranquilizer.
- Teeth grinding at night.

- Abnormal growth or rickets in children.
- Osteoporosis in adults.
- Convulsions.
- Cramps, muscle spasms, twitching.
- Heartbeat irregularities.
- Allergies.
- Bleeding tendencies.

[] [] [] [] [] []

UNDERSTANDING CALCIUM ABSORPTION

1. **Exercise** is an *ESSENTIAL* part of calcium absorption. Rapid loss of calcium due to inactivity contributes to exhaustion in bedridden people. Space program tests showed calcium loss in weightlessness, regardless of calcium in their food, or supplements. However, there is also calcium loss during sustained over-vigorous exercise.

2. **Excessive mental, emotional, or physical stress** causes excretion of calcium to be greater, regardless of the amount of intake. Stress management becomes a critical part of health.

3. **Hydrochloric acid** is *NECESSARY* in your stomach for proper calcium absorption. On the other hand, calcium cannot be absorbed in a system that is too acidic, **so pH balance is critical.**

4. **Normal levels of estrogen or testosterone** are necessary to absorb calcium. Aging encourages calcium deficiency because of generally low hormone levels.

> *Your doctor can check your hormone levels though a blood test. You may not know that low* ***estrogen*** *can cause cellular changes that cause irritation when urinating for women, and symptoms*

*can be mistaken for a bladder infection. You also
may not know that low **testosterone** is a cause of low
sex drive in both men and women. It is also
important to know that to protect against
osteoporosis you need **progesterone** to build bone.
Health food stores carry natural herbs, and
hormone products, that do not have side effects like
those you could get from drug hormone
replacements.*

5. **Drugs** have varying effects on calcium absorption.
    Some (like antibiotics) increase the body's need for
    calcium, and some (like steroids) decrease absorption.
    Antibiotics destroy beneficial intestinal bacteria needed
    for calcium absorption. Following antibiotics, always
    re-establish healthy intestinal flora with friendly bacteria
    products from the health food stores. Take two to three
    times the recommended dose for 2 months.

6. **Phytic acid and oxalates** in certain foods such as grains,
    all legumes, rhubarb, potatoes, cauliflower, broccoli,
    spinach and asparagus hinder calcium absorption, unless
    cooked, steamed or sprouted.

7. **Vitamin F (essential fatty acids)** is needed for calcium
    absorption. Use cold-pressed oils, whole grains, and
    unprocessed nuts and seeds; or consider supplements
    like Flaxseed, Black-Currant Seed, Hemp, Borage oil, or
    Emu oil.

8. **Vitamin D** has a potent effect on intestinal absorption of
    calcium. Too many food products and supplements
    fortified with Vitamin D, and high intake of eggs and
    fish, can cause too much calcium absorption. THERE IS
    THAT WORD MODERATION AGAIN! Ultra-violet
    light in sunlight on the skin, changes a form of
    cholesterol to Vitamin D. You need about 30 minutes
    per day of sunlight for vitamin D synthesis. But, you

254

can soak up Vitamin D all day and still be deficient, if you are not getting enough Vitamin A and Vitamin C.

9. **Phosphorus** is needed to absorb calcium; too much phosphorus will cause calcium loss, as excess phosphorus leaves the body as calcium phosphate. We have a high phosphorus diet in this country with red meat, cereal, dairy, and carbonated drinks. Many children and adults have cereal as a major component of their diet.

10. **Sodium fluoride** used by drug companies and the dental profession is a calcium antagonist. Calcium fluoride is safer. You can buy calcium fluoride cell salts in health food stores.

11. **Abnormal fluid consumption, use of prescription or herbal diuretics** can flush minerals out through your kidneys. Drink fluids regularly throughout the day, rather than large amounts at one time. Never lose sight of finding the *cause* of symptoms now, rather than treating chronic symptoms for a lifetime.

12. **Diarrhea** can cause loss of nutrients. It is important to evaluate food allergies, poor digestion of milk sugar, and alternating constipation and diarrhea. A colon cleanse could perform miracles. BioPlasma cell salts may be very helpful in correcting chronic diarrhea.

13. **White sugar** depletes calcium because it drives out calcium, and shifts body chemistry in ways that can cause many health problems.

14. **Inherited weaknesses** are becoming more prominent each generation. Seemingly healthy children are born with toxic conditions, nutritional deficiencies, and allergies.

15. **Magnesium** is calcium's co-pilot. Most anti-aging daily supplement programs will recommend magnesium and potassium supplements. Magnesium makes urine more solvent to hold crystals in solution, for people who are prone to calcium oxalate *kidney stones*, or *gallstones*. It is doubtful you are getting enough magnesium unless you eat plenty of raw and unprocessed foods, because magnesium is extremely sensitive to heat.

16. **Commercial frozen vegetables** may contain EDTA, and this agent partially removes zinc, manganese, and calcium. Frozen vegetables in a health food store will not contain EDTA.

17. **Too high fiber diet** can cause anywhere from 100-400 milligrams of calcium to be lost per day. *MODERATION IN EVERYTHING!!!*

18. **A high protein diet** contributes to low calcium levels, because it increases the body's need for calcium, to neutralize acid conditions produced by excess protein. *MODERATION AGAIN!!!* This is very important in light of the current trend towards high protein diets.

19. **Vitamin K** produces a protein that attracts calcium into bone tissues. Vitamin K is poorly produced in an unhealthy intestine that has micro-organism overgrowth, low healthy bacteria, and cellular dehydration. *Another reason for drinking your correct amount of water daily!*

20. **Boron**, a trace mineral long considered not essential to nutrition, is now indicated as reducing calcium loss. Some calcium supplements do contain boron, but you can get ample boron by eating pears, apples, grapes, leafy vegetables, nuts, and legumes.

21. **Alcohol, caffeine, and smoking** interfere with calcium absorption.

22. **Trace minerals** enhance absorption, metabolism and utilization of calcium. Vegetables grown on commercial land no longer contain the trace minerals found in those same vegetables, when Grandma raised and ate them.

23. **Thyroid disorders** can cause calcium loss. *Check your thyroid activity at home with this method* **ONCE A MONTH***:*

    - *With a digital or mercury thermometer, check your oral temperature after you have been up for several hours,* **three times each day, for three days.** *You do not have to be sedentary, but you should not take your temperatures immediately after exercise. Take oral temperatures at least 15 minutes after food or drink. A digital thermometer will beep in about 30 seconds; a mercury thermometer takes three to four minutes. The old fashion mercury thermometer (also available in non-mercury) may take longer, but may be more accurate. Many people have reported to me that their ear and digital thermometers can give low, or back to back different readings.*

    - *Women with menstrual cycles start on day two of the flow.*

    - *Individual "normal" readings may vary slightly, but temperatures* **less than** *98.4 F or* **above** *98.6 F orally are outside of a normal range. If readings are low, increase vegetables for more potassium. Consider one to two cayenne pepper (40,000 heat unit strength) in vegicaps two to three times a day,* **always with food.** *Most people stop feeling stomach warmth with cayenne after several weeks. If temperatures do not improve, get a thyroid*

257

evaluation by your doctor, and ask him or her to evaluate reverse T3.

The thyroid is responsible for regulating the rate at which all of your metabolic processes proceed. If the gland's output of thyroid hormone drops, blood tests will reflect the decrease. There is another problem that is a part of medical training, but still not a practicing option by most physicians. You could suffer from the effects even if the thyroid gland itself tests normal. You can have the symptoms associated with the problem even if you are taking thyroid medication. This second route to thyroid function failure takes place **outside** the gland. To have an optimal working of the thyroid *system*, the body must convert most of the hormone the thyroid secretes, called T4, into a compound called T3. **Under prolonged stress, your body might start producing the wrong kind of T3,** and convert T4 into *reverse* T3, which is biologically inert. Reverse T3 is the mirror image of T3, yet it has no biological activity. By replacing some of the prescribed T4 with **time-release** T3, the reverse T3 gets displaced by active T3, and metabolism may return to normal.

Body temperature is the most reliable way to determine thyroid **activity**. The farther below the normal 98.6 F orally you are, the more likely your thyroid activity is below par. If the temperatures are erratic up and down, it can be an indication of adrenal stress. Dr. E. Denis Wilson, who deserves credit for fully developing this revolutionary concept, called it Wilson's Syndrome. Most Doctors are not familiar enough with **Wilson's Syndrome** to effectively treat the problem. For more information contact the Center for Natural Medicine, in Portland, Oregon. Contact information is listed in the

Resource References. Also check the internet for information on Wilson's Syndrome.

TO STRENGTHEN A SLUGGISH THYROID WITH NATURAL METHODS:

- *Consider kelp, three-five tablets three times a day; use seaweeds in soups and stews. Kelp supplies B12 for the vegetarian; absorbs elements from the sea that almost completely mirror human blood in amino acids, minerals and trace elements.*

- *Eat fish at least three times a week.*

- *Consider 400-800 I.U. of **dry** Vitamin E daily to stimulate the pituitary gland, which stimulates the thyroid. Exercise daily to activate the hypothalamus, that activates the pituitary. You can also consider Vitex, an herb that regulates the pituitary. The body is an interrelated system!*

- *Consider alive food supplements listed in the Digestion chapter.*

- *Use cold-pressed oils high in essential fatty acids that produce prostaglandins, needed for hormone and enzyme production. Do not consume refined oils. Unrefined oils are currently sold mostly in health food stores.*

- *Avoid caffeine and smoking because they encourage the intake of sweets that overstress the thyroid.*

- *Consume low simple carbohydrates: no refined sugar, fruit juice (unless diluted in half), dried fruit (unless in very small amounts), or refined grains. Use natural sugars in small amounts; fresh fruit once or twice a day only. Simple sugars in excess can stress the thyroid, and cause people to gain weight in their abdomen, hips, and thighs. Increase complex carbohydrates such as whole grains, potatoes, starchy vegetables and legumes.*

- *Eliminate chlorine in water and bathing, as chlorine shuts down thyroid function by preventing absorption of iodine and the amino acid thyrosine.*

- *Reduce **excessive** use of soy protein that can weaken thyroid function.*

[] [] [] [] [] []

THE ONLY SOURCE OF CALCIUM IS NOT FROM THE COW!

The recommended daily allowance of calcium is set at 800-1000 milligrams; 1200-1500 milligrams per day for post-menopausal women; 400-800 milligrams per day for children. Stress and exercise levels influence how much calcium you need, and how well it is absorbed.

The dairy association has persuaded us that milk is the best source of calcium, but it is only <u>one</u> source. Many foods with fewer digestive, mucus forming, and allergic symptoms, plus lower in phosphorus than dairy are also **excellent** sources of calcium.

Another problem with dairy products is strontium 90. It is a radioactive substance placed into the clouds by nuclear activity in some areas, absorbed by the grass from rain, eaten by the cows, and accepted by their

*mammary glands; then we drink the milk. The strontium
90 is accepted in the bones like calcium, and may
contribute to the cause of some bone cancers. Bone
meal from animals can also have strontium 90, so it is
not a recommended source of calcium.* **USE DAIRY
PRODUCTS FOR SOCIAL FOOD, AND NOT A
SOURCE OF CALCIUM.**

Dolomite is ground rock, and not recommended with the
better absorbed chelated minerals available. Tums is advertised
as a source of calcium. Two tablets are very low in biologically
available calcium, and contains mineral oil and talc. Beware that
commercials can recommend products that mask a much more
serious problem. Dehydration or pH imbalance is a must
consideration if you have an upset stomach, symptoms of poor
digestion, or you are concerned about calcium absorption.

Four main types of calcium: calcium lactate is the same type
found in milk; calcium gluconate (a salt from gluconic acid
prepared by the oxidation of glucose) is easy to digest, but like
calcium lactate, takes a large quantity to get enough daily;
*calcium carbonate (a salt of carbonic acid formed in solution by
carbon dioxide in water) is from lime used in making cement, so
this poorly absorbed form of calcium is not recommended.*
Calcium citrate is bound to lemon fruit acids, and easier for the
body to absorb and utilize. Regardless of the source of calcium,
a major consideration is Vitamin D3, the essential hormonal
form of Vitamin D, without which calcium cannot be used by the
body for bone formation. Look for D3 in your calcium
supplements.

If you ROTATE all healthy foods, you are likely to consume
many sources of calcium: *Rotate the following:*

Seeds (especially sesame), broccoli, cabbage,
cauliflower, radish, blackstrap molasses, maple syrup,
sardines, salmon, tuna, nuts (especially almond),
soybeans, peanuts, green leaf and stalk vegetables, egg
yolk, carob, shellfish and fish, asparagus, buckwheat,
whole grains, tomato, potato, carrots, and figs. Eating

261

sea vegetables four times a week will provide quality calcium if you do not eat dairy products. There are many varieties of seaweeds in health food stores that greatly improve the nutrition of many recipes. **IN OTHER WORDS, EAT A WIDE VARIETY OF WHOLE GRAINS AND FRESH UNPROCESSED FOODS, AND YOU WILL GET YOUR CALCIUM, PLUS A WHOLE LOT MORE!!!**

[] [] [] [] [] []

YOUR LYMPHATIC SYSTEM

You cannot talk body wellness without understanding there is more circulating in your body than just blood. The lymphatic system is less understood, yet there is twice as much lymph in the body as there is blood, and twice as many lymphatic vessels as there are blood vessels. The lymph system protects your health.

Did you ever pop a blister and notice the clear liquid inside? This is lymph, a yellowish fluid that is "squeezed" throughout the body in its own private circulation system. The lymph system is a vast system like the blood vessels, with one big difference ... it has no heart to keep it moving. The lymph vessels are squeezed, and lymph pushed along and filtered through lymph nodes, by deep breathing and specific exercises.

> *The best activity for the lymphatic system is any BOUNCING action previously discussed, or stroking of any discomfort area towards the chest. It is alright to choose an exercise two to three days a week for circulatory health, or exercise that strengthens muscle tone. Those exercise options should be in addition to exercise for 15 minutes* **DAILY** *to move the lymph.*

As blood circulates and exchanges nutrients and hormones for waste products, it leaks fluids. These fluids must return to the blood, but first they are filtered through lymph nodes.

262

ANYTIME THE LYMPH BACKS UP YOU CAN EXPERIENCE PHYSICAL SYMPTOMS!!! A clogged lymph system can mean upper respiratory infections, sinus or ear infections, throat problems, colds, tonsillitis as well as bronchitis and pneumonia, low back ache, pain anywhere, and tissue swelling. We need to keep the lymph system moving, and one way is through **THE RIGHT CHOICE OF EXERCISE.**

OTHER WAYS TO CARE FOR YOUR LYMPHATIC SYSTEM

- **Consume the best water** you can find in the amount specific for your body weight daily, which is one ounce of water for each two pounds of body weight. For many people who are overweight, the maximum will be 12-16 glasses (three to four quarts) of water because of the time limit in a day, so if your needs are over that, make sure you get *at least* that much.

- **Reduce dietary fats** that can clog systems anywhere in the body; *but you do need essential fatty acids.* Eliminate refined grains and oils, and eat more raw or dry roasted nuts and seeds.

- **Blood cleansing formulas** help clear out both toxic blood and toxic lymph conditions. Herbs like echinacea, goldenseal, capsicum, licorice root, hawthorn berries, ginger, and fenugreek tea all help strengthen and clear this extensive network. Unrefined Aloe Vera is an **exceptional** blood and lymph cleanser.

- **Liquid chlorophyll, Spirulina, Blue-Green Algae, wheat or barley grass,** are also good blood and lymph system cleansers.

- **Eat fresh fruits *in moderation* and lots of raw vegetables.** Organic fruits and vegetables are always

263

recommended because of more natural nutritional content, and less chemicals.

-   **Stimulate lymphatic drainage** *in the following ways:*

    1. Located at the bottom part of the breast bone is a reflex point. Vigorously rub that area for two minutes to help lymphatic drainage. This is the collection area for lymph drainage coming from the head down, or up from the feet.

    2. Start under the jaw and "milk" the big muscle down the throat on each side of the neck, *TOWARDS THE HEART.*

    3. Start just behind the ears and "milk" downward towards the shoulders. Each time move closer toward the spinal column. This can relieve headaches, and muscle tension.

    4. Fast stroke in any area that is symptomatic, seven-ten times towards the heart every 10-15 minutes until relief occurs. This, or any of the above suggestions may not be appropriate for some medical conditions. If you are in doubt, ask your doctor.

HOW YOUR LYMPHATIC SYSTEM PROTECTS YOUR HEALTH

Your cells are constantly in the process of taking in nutrients and eliminating toxic wastes through the following series of events:

-   Through the capillaries flow blood that is 91 percent water, oxygen, nutrients, and three blood proteins (albumin, globulin, and fibrinogen). The blood proteins hold the water in the capillaries, as the oxygen and nutrients go through tiny pores to nourish the nearby tightly packed cells.

- White blood cells circulate among those packed cells protecting you from bacteria and viruses, and the lymphatic system carries away any remaining toxins and wastes.

IN THIS PERFECTLY FUNCTIONING SYSTEM, YOUR HEALTH IS MAINTAINED AND PROTECTED. SO, WHY ARE SO MANY PEOPLE STRUGGLING WITH HEALTH?

- The pores in the capillaries become **enlarged** from drugs and/or stress. Drugs are being used in epidemic proportions. Even if you do not take any drugs, no one in modern America can escape stress. Stress can come from emotional, financial, relationship or career issues; polluted electromagnetic frequencies in the atmosphere; total chemical environment; nutritional imbalances, dehydration, or build up of toxic wastes in the body. Stress from any cause, allows the smallest of the blood proteins (albumin) to pass through the enlarged capillary pores. With albumin's magnetic attraction to water, the water is pulled out of the capillaries, and surround the cells. Cells, separated with proteins and water, are unable to correctly receive oxygen and nutrients. This is the beginning of degenerative changes in the cells that can lead to symptoms and disease.

- A slow moving lymphatic system is not able to keep up with pulling off the water and proteins. When this condition builds up in any body area, you can experience *local* symptoms.

HOW DO YOU PROTECT YOUR LYMPHATICS?

1. Use drugs only in an acute, emergency, or a medical conditions when nothing else will protect your health or life. IF YOU NEED DRUGS, YOU ALSO NEED THE "LAWS" OF WELLNESS TO HELP YOUR BODY HEAL!

2. Learn how to cope with daily stress and build self-esteem.

3. Drink your maximum amount of water daily, *unless otherwise indicated by an existing medical condition.*

4. Do "bouncing" type exercise 15 minutes once or twice daily. This means coming down on the bottom of your feet as you exercise, like in walking, as opposed to riding a bike. If you cannot exercise, sit in a chair with your feet on a trampoline, and have someone else do the jumping. The vibration will help move the lymph.

5. Protect your liver and lymphatic system with regular cleansing recommendations made in the Elimination chapter.

6. Read the book *THE GOLDEN SEVEN PLUS ONE,* by C. Samuel West. I found it very helpful on lymphatic exercise, and cellular health (refer to Resource References).

[] [] [] [] [] []

ANOTHER FORM OF ENERGY - MAGNETISM

As a health "student," one value you should get from this book is exposure to many different subjects that affect health. Our modern society has polluted or reduced our exposure to the natural balance of nature. THE AVERAGE PERSON IS LOW IN ENVIRONMENTAL ELECTROMAGNETIC INTAKE DUE TO THE EARTH'S MAGNETIC FIELD BEING

POLLUTED. POWER LINES, TELEVISION, MICROWAVES, RADAR, CELL PHONES, BEEPERS, FLOURESCENT LIGHTS, MODERN LIVING IN STEEL BUILDINGS, CARS, PLANES, TRAINS, BUSES, AND SUBWAYS ARE JUST SOME EXAMPLES THAT DEPRIVE US OF REGULAR EXPOSURE TO OUR NATURAL ENVIRONMENT.

Every atom, molecule, cell, tissue and organ in our body resonates, or vibrates at its own particular frequency. That body frequency NATURALLY vibrates to, and connects with the earth's energy. This *combination* of energy can occur in every cell, organ and system of our body. It alters the rate of cellular activity, and the chemical processes that effect overall changes in our body.

The same body effects can be "created" by *applying* a magnetic field which performs in the same way. It only takes a very low intensity magnetic field to effect chemical reactions that have a biological effect on our body.

There are two main types of magnetism:

-   *A temporary magnetic field puts out a magnetic field only while electricity is flowing through coils of wire by continually reversing the poles. Changing the direction of a magnetic field induces an electromagnetic force (EMF), producing electrical energy. This can cause cellular chaos, and can create problems as we surround our lives with more and more electrical products. This is why you will read articles on not sleeping with electric blankets, or on heated waterbeds.*

-   *Permanent magnetism follows a continuous closed path which travels from North pole to South pole. This is not hazardous because the magnetic field does not change ... North and South do not reverse positions causing chaos. Magnetic therapy is a respected medical approach elsewhere in the world,*

267

but this country concentrates on more profitable drugs and surgery. The noticeable value of improved circulation with permanent magnetism could benefit situations like sleep problems, pain, stiffness, and injury. Any effort to improve circulation is a "first do no harm" approach to symptoms worth checking out.

SOME ENERGY YOU DO NOT WANT!

We cannot change our technological world. However, we can no longer be *unaware* of the health risks associated with modern lifestyles. The rapid changes in our natural environment with all the advancements of electrical industrialization, have created energy changes that directly affect us on all levels of mental, emotional, and physical. Our natural frequency range is constantly being hit by man-made frequencies. Water is within the natural frequency range. That is why a hot shower or bath is so soothing and relaxing to the body. As water envelops the body, it cleans away the surrounding higher frequencies, and brings it back in resonance with the earth's average frequency range. Another reason for taking a relaxing shower or bath before going to bed.

Man and all species must adapt to their environment or die. Sometimes it may take a species thousands of years to adapt. Sometimes the species may die out before it can adapt to changes in the environment. Our bodies lived in harmony with the earth's natural frequency before electricity. We need to better understand the role frequencies play in our natural environment. Our only hope is to figure a way to detect, protect and limit the impact modern technology has on the human body. We can no longer survive without electricity … and we can no longer survive *unhurt* in this rapidly polluted environment. We must strive to limit any adverse impact modern technology has on our health and well being.

The magnetic field of the human brain and the earth's normal magnetic beat are very similar. When something accelerates, or slows the brain's normal magnetic beat, it can affect the body by making us excited or drowsy. You cannot see, hear, smell, or taste electromagnetic waves that are assaulting you everyday. Electrical equipment produces frequencies in a range that is destructive to biological systems, including the body's *natural* electrical balance. *It could be the difference between health or chronic illness, to check on ways to protect yourself and/or your loved ones in our electromagnetic polluted environment.*

[] [] [] [] [] []

THE POWER TO HEAL and other health books are part of the exciting adventure in learning about personal development on all levels of spiritual, mental, emotional, and physical. This book is meant to *introduce* you to different subjects of wellness. Now you have a basis to start your health journey ... **a foundation on which to grow on all levels of spiritual, mental, emotional, and physical.** You will be adding to your knowledge the rest of your life ... *one day at a time.*

This is the day which the Lord hath made. We will rejoice and be glad in it.

Psalms 118, 24

To achieve optimum health means understanding about supplements ... so to complete your well-rounded course in wellness, I encourage you to read on ...

CHAPTER 6

SUPPLEMENT GUIDANCE

Have you ever gone into a health food store and become thoroughly confused as to what supplements to buy? Too often the store staff you rely on to give you helpful and correct information are speaking from such limited knowledge, that you are likely not to receive the health benefits you expect. This can be costly, and discouraging, and has been proven over and over in my practice, as very ill clients bring in their "bags" of supplements.

We are all bio-chemically different, with different hereditary factors. In addition, a hard working farmer, who is able to pay his bills, has a loving wife and happy children, and eats his organically raised food, varies a lot from a city salesman who struggles with bills, has marital and child problems, and eats mostly fast foods. Add to that all the social stresses, surgery, existing disease state, inactivity, air pollution, water contamination, aging, food chemicals, electromagnetic polluted frequencies, positive and negative ion imbalance, and medications, makes it impossible to have standards of health for everyone based on any "normal values." Acknowledging current stress levels, what nutritional needs you had in the past, may be different than what you need today.

All the variables that make up a person's nutritional needs are unique to that individual "alone." If you had 100 people in a room, they would all have different nutritional needs, so taking the **same** multi-vitamin and mineral supplement would create *some imbalances in everyone*! The theory is you would excrete what you do not need ... *but at what price to body stress? People can get an initial energy boost from a multiple supplement, but as their body catches up on nutrients, they continue to take the same formula in amounts they **now do not need**!!!* I have a constant flow of people in my office saying they are taking supplements they thought helped at first, but now they do not feel well. **This is why I only recommend alive food**

supplements *that act like food in the body, and not drugs.* **STAY WITH WHOLE FOOD SUPPLEMENTS ... DO NOT PLAY GUESSING GAMES WITH YOUR BODY!!! YOU MAY BE CREATING MORE PROBLEMS THAN YOU ARE TRYING TO RESOLVE!**

WE CANNOT CONSUME THE AMOUNT OF FOOD WE NEED TO KEEP UP WITH THE MANY STRESSES IN OUR SOCIETY. Today's meals do not even begin to compare with the quality of food our grandparents ate. *The following information is in MEGA NUTRITION by Richard Kunin M.D:*

WAYS NUTRITIONAL VALUES CAN BE ALTERED:

- Over the years our soil has changed in mineral content. The addition of chemicals and insecticides instead of nutritional replacement, plus transporting to the store, storage there and in your home cost our food about 20% of its nutritional value.

- A large portion of the American diet is, or has been frozen, costing about 5% of the nutritional value. Another 5% is lost in washing or peeling fruits and vegetables.

- Cooking conservatively reduces nutritional value by 20%.

- Chemical preservatives, additives, sweeteners, etc. in processed food that has risen from 10% in 1940 to presently over 60% greatly affects nutritional value. We are left with getting far fewer nutrients than our grandparents got from the same food.

- Laboratory studies show people who subsist on refined, processed, and canned food (which makes up 60% of the American diet) will not be provided with adequate nutrition. Since the American diet is

271

too often as high as 45% fat, and 25% sugar, this leaves 30% of the diet to provide the nutrients vital to health and well being. With all the previously mentioned facts robbing that 30%, it is estimated too many people have their health protected by only a small portion of their food intake.

Even more alarming is that all the above does not take into consideration correct digestion, absorption, and metabolism. *The end value of our food is very scary,* considering sales volumes of antacids, laxatives, and Tagamet (reached the #1 drug sales in the world), and children now as chronically and acutely ill as adults.

[] [] [] [] [] []

IN MODERN SOCIETY WE MUST CONSIDER "CORRECT" SUPPLEMENTATION TO OUR DIET TO GET OUR NUTRUITIONAL NEEDS. SO, **WHAT MAKES A CERTAIN VITAMIN CHOICE A GOOD CHOICE?**

This paragraph from THE NATIONAL ACADEMY OF RESEARCH BIOCHEMISTS newsletter states:

"One of the most perilous deceptions of those who place pesos above principles is the passing off on a gullible public, phony, synthetic vitamins or crystalline-pure fractions of vitamin complexes and ballyhooing that the body does not know the difference. That phrase was coined on the one and only Madison Avenue, where truth is spelled MONEY. At the very best, synthetic or pure vitamin fractions can function in the human body as only a drug or pharmaceutical agent ... certainly not as a physiological supporting nutrient. At worse, the counterfeit supplements can seriously impair the most important of body functions by contributing to biochemical imbalance. Synthetic vitamins are **MIRROR IMAGES** *of natural vitamins. However, keep*

272

in mind that synthetic vitamins are not vitamins at all but synthesized FRACTIONS of a vitamin complex, a mirror image duplicate of just a portion of the real, biologically active nutritional complex. There is no possible way that a fraction of a vitamin be called a vitamin. The analogy here is essentially the same as an automobile salesman handing you a wheel from a car and telling you the wheel is the whole automobile."

In nature and in the body, vitamins are found in combination with other factors. An extracted vitamin may be "structurally" identical to a "part" of the whole, but the biologic and functional role of the "whole" form will be different acting in concert with many other factors. *Imbalance can be produced by well meaning health enthusiasts, trying to balance the system without enough information about their specific body needs.* Do not "THINK ZINC" just because an article listed some of your symptoms, and zinc helped the author. *Why are you not absorbing zinc, is a more important problem, than the fact you are low in zinc.*

The nutrient amount that would keep a person well who has always been healthy, may vary enormously with the amount needed for a person who has had many years of illness and drug therapy. If supplement fractions are considered, it should be only after medical determination shows a need for that particular fraction. **Supplement choices should always reflect a bond with nature.**

Vitamins by themselves cannot prevent or correct a deficiency. It is important to combine them with proteins, fatty acids, minerals, and enzymes which the body needs to use them efficiently. Take vitamins with meals, but *never lose sight of the ultimate goal to heal the organs of digestion, so you get the MOST from the quality food you eat, or the supplements you take. Trace minerals, pH balance, water, essential fatty acids, and controlled Candida yeast and parasites, are all elements in digestion evaluation.*

273

[] [] [] [] [] []

LET'S PUT INTO PERSPECTIVE THE
THREAT OF GETTING TOO MANY VITAMINS.

Every year countless of people are poisoned by some drug, which can be bought casually over the counter. Others sicken or die from overdoses of sleeping drugs or tranquilizers. Hospitals are full of patients suffering from some disorder brought on by some medication their doctor is giving them. Every advertisement for pharmaceutical drugs, which appears in medical journals, must carry a long list of possible harmful side effects. And, the side effects list is very frightening indeed! *Drugs are poison, and that is why you need a prescription, so you can be carefully monitored.*

In the future you will hear a lot of politically motivated comments about the harmful side effects of too many vitamins. *It will draw your attention away from the REAL issues at hand...the over-medication of people, the needless surgery, the thousands of worthless drugs, the poor statistics on health results, the deterioration of health in our country, and the effort that is being made to prevent people from being PART OF THEIR OWN MEDICAL TREATMENT PLAN.*

DISEASE ... NOT HEALTH ... IS BIG BUSINESS!!!

My mother died at age 34 from leucopenia (low white blood count). Her death was a suspected result of taking long term use of an over the counter drug for pain relief from headaches, muscle and joint pain. Even though the flyers in drug packaging gives harmful side effects, WHO READS IT? OR IF THEY DO, WHO PAYS ANY ATTENTION TO IT IF THEY THINK IT WILL HELP? As a society we seem willing to take drugs with serious side effects, but become unbelievably cautious when the subject of vitamins is discussed, *because the doctors are dispensing drugs, not discussing supplements.* A compassionate doctor who spent years learning the immense field of medicine has helped all of us at one time or another. Too

274

often, nutrition and the principles of "wellness" are largely ignored by the medical profession, concentrating on what he or she knows about crisis medicine.

Many foreign countries are years ahead of the United States in making health products, and anti-aging techniques readily available to their people. The importance of parasite control is accepted preventive medicine in some countries. I have had clients from the Caribbean and Australia who are use to buying readily available parasite products routinely. On arrival in this country, one man from Australia asked a pharmacist where to find the parasite products, and was sent to the pet department. We need to take as good care of the people in this country, as we do our animals.

We do need to take supplements with knowledge, but the damage from supplement abuse does not BEGIN to compare to the damage from drug abuse. The more you understand the **balance** of whole food nutrients, rather than FRACTIONS that chemically look like a portion of the whole complex, the less likely you are to take supplements *you do not need. Separating the single nutrient from the whole, like single vitamins, minerals, or amino acids, can cause a problem in the body balance.* If you consider any supplement, you should have some understanding of that product meeting your specific needs, the "wholeness" with nature, and the absorption quality of the choice.

It should be noted here that there could be a danger in taking too many supplements that contain *all* the trace minerals. My experience has shown that regardless of sex or size, there is a definite difference in the tolerance level of taking up to three supplements with *all* the trace minerals, and taking four or more. Three supplements containing all the trace minerals consistently tested well on my Biofeedback equipment, but four consistently tested as being too much, for all people tested. The body may handle short-term excess, but long term excess could be destructive as the body struggles to get rid of nutrients you do not need. *Remember, they are called "trace" minerals, not "unlimited" minerals! Too much of a good thing does not make it better.*

[] [] [] [] [] []

YOU SHOULD BE AWARE OF THE FOLLOWING WHEN YOU ARE TAKING SUPPLEMENTS:

- All vitamins are not created equally. Examples of "true" natural supplements are seaweed or algae, wheat grass, barley green, bee pollen, green tea, or aloe vera.

- *COMMERCIAL SUPPLEMENTS MAY VARY CONSIDERABLY, SO YOU NEED TO STICK WITH COMPANIES THAT MAINTAIN THE HIGHEST QUALITY. That does not mean the company with fancy advertisement, or an enthusiastic sales person will necessarily recommend what is best for "you." We are all biochemically different. Few people can test what they take on Biofeedback equipment available in practitioner's offices. It would be advisable for anyone taking supplements to buy a book on Biokinesiology. Testing a supplement using arm or finger strength can be learned by anyone, and can be very helpful in making supplement choices.*

ANY OF THE FOLLOWING STANDARDS MAY VARY WITH DIFFERENT COMPANIES:

- *Full vitamin potency* listed on the label does not have to be in the product when shipped.

- If not manufactured correctly, vitamins can be much weaker than the label claims by the time you purchase that product.

- Manufacturers are not required to prove that their product lasts for an extended period of time.

- A quality control lab is not required in a vitamin manufacturing facility. KNOW YOUR COMPANY ...

276

DO NOT BARGAIN SHOP!!! BUY THE BEST SUPPLEMENTS, AND TRUST YOUR CHOSEN COMPANY TO GIVE YOU THE QUALITY YOU DESERVE. For example, not all "Echinacea" is the same extracted potency. The therapeutic strength can be shockingly low. When you get good advice about proven high quality supplements, it is worth serious consideration.

This comment from Dr. Julian Whitaker M.D.'S WELLNESS JOURNAL, January 1, 2000 states, *"For millions of people, the vitamin craze has become a cruel hoax. Too many vitamin peddlers have swamped the marketplace, making outlandish claims and pushing questionable pills with one dominant motive – to make a fast buck at the expense of your health."* He continues to say, *"I see so many people taking vitamins by the fistful, but they're NOT getting well. The problem is you're not absorbing many of the vitamins you're swallowing. You're wasting a lot of money on pills that will do you no good ... and may even be triggering the very conditions you're trying to prevent!"*

[] [] [] [] [] []

IN YOUR EFFORT TO ASSUME SELF-RESPONSIBILITY FOR YOUR HEALTH, YOU MAY ASK, "WHERE DO I START?"

- **Eliminate many of the over-the-counter drugs** in your medicine cabinet. Any one of them can possibly cause more illness than they treat. ALWAYS FIND OUT WHY YOU HAVE A SYMPTOM INSTEAD OF JUST TRYING TO SUPPRESS THE SYMPTOM!!! You do need first aid supplies, but many times those crisis situations are actually "chronic" symptoms that got worse.

- **Use drugs only under the direction of a medical doctor**. INSIST on his assurance that nothing else will do. If your doctor is traditional in his practice, all appropriate tests are normal, and he or she does not support your interest in finding the CAUSE of your problems, consider a second opinion from an alternative practitioner. Ultimately only you are responsible for your health. No one else cares as much as you.

- **LEARN TO BE AWARE OF BODY LANGUAGE.** *PAIN AND DISCOMFORT IS THE BODY TRYING TO TELL YOU SOMETHING! IT IS A LOT EASIER TO TURN YOUR HEALTH AROUND WITH THE FIRST SYMPTOM THAN TO TREAT ESTABLISHED DISEASE!!!*

- **Understanding your "health" is a lifetime of continuing education** on all levels of spiritual, mental, emotional, and physical. Your health education should be a "hobby" of endurance, learning from *many* teachers of wellness. This path will give your life new purpose and rewards, as you journey towards optimum health. Accept your health education as a gift, and be proud of taking responsibility for your health.

- **Check your newspapers or other local service resources for health expos.** Expos allow you to talk to a variety of health oriented practitioners, and listen to professionals teaching about wellness.

[] [] [] [] [] []

CONGRATULATIONS TO THOSE WHO HAVE COMPLETED THE LAST SIX CHAPTERS.

THIS QUOTE BY AN UNKNOWN WRITER MAY FIT THE WAY YOU FEEL:

"WE HAVE NOT SUCCEEDED IN ANSWERING ALL YOUR PROBLEMS. THE ANSWERS WE HAVE FOUND ONLY SERVE TO RAISE A WHOLE SET OF NEW QUESTIONS. IN SOME WAYS WE FEEL WE ARE CONFUSED ON A HIGHER LEVEL, BUT ABOUT MORE IMPORTANT THINGS."

THE ROAD TO HEALTH BECOMES EASIER
THROUGH EDUCATION

... read on for a few final comments ...

SUMMARY

THE POWER OF HEALING ... A METAMORPHOSIS
THE NEW "YOU" EMERGES

"... let us run with endurance the race that is set before us."

Hebrews 12:1

YOU are responsible for your well being. WELLNESS is as much a state of mind, as it is being free of disease. As you live by health promoting standards, the frustrations of life that may once have seemed overwhelming, can now be dealt with as minor annoyances. You have now achieved the ability to control your health, rather than be controlled by your illnesses.

For me, graduation from the "school of health" was the day I climbed to 9,795-foot Eagle Cap Peak in northeastern Oregon. The 40 miles I hiked in six days would have been achievement enough considering my medical history. However, climbing a mountain that just a few years earlier seemed an impossible dream, became an exhilarating highlight in my life. If I could do that hike ... what else could I do? Each accomplishment produced the energy needed to stretch into new directions ... with new goals ... and new hope for the future.

[] [] [] [] [] []

Being a health success story can be another kind of challenge ... in communication. You have all you can handle learning and applying new knowledge to improve YOUR health, so do not take on the health problems of people around you. Most people do not appreciate being told that what is helping you will also be the best thing for them. *ONLY* when they are motivated because of their own illness, or are impressed by your good health, will they be willing to make different choices in their lives. Take care of your own health ... teach through

280

EXAMPLE! People want to listen when they *ask* what you are doing to improve your health.

Not everyone is willing or able to be strict with his or her health routine all the time. MODERATION is the key! If you do not have adverse reactions, you may choose to occasionally enjoy a treat socially that is not a perfect health recommendation. Sensible social treats may keep you from feeling deprived, and keep you health-oriented at other times. Remember that **you make or break your health at home**, where you should eat most of your meals. If you eat out a lot, learn to be more selective, and take alive food supplements.

Heredity and aging get the blame for far too much illness today. Many problems are self-inflicted through overhydration or underhydration, poor dietary and habit choices, and through overzealous supplement efforts that create body imbalances. When you have symptoms, realize your body is telling you there are problems. Learn to *TUNE IN TO BODY LANGUAGE.* Access how your symptoms may be presently due to neglecting one or more of the "LAWS" OF WELLNESS. As you make changes, and your health improves, you will gain confidence from the miracles that can be experienced through your efforts. You will want to expand your knowledge to support health naturally. *Learning ways to protect your health so you feel well each day, becomes your new hobby.*

Your new hobby is not without challenges. Every health suggestion that comes out in print is enthusiastically presented as *the answer* in achieving wellness. Conflicting opinions in many books concentrating on one aspect of health at the expense of the whole, and a fever for detailed options have led to confusion and frustration. It is understandable why some people refuse to get involved with their own health management. When we do make a choice, it often is oversimplified from reading an article like *THINK ZINC.* It does not follow that all you have to do for wellness is to take zinc supplements. Relying solely on your doctor to deal with chronic illness is not the answer either. The answer lies in BALANCE. Live by the COMMON SENSE laws that allow the body to work at optimum performance, or heal itself if possible. Our new and improved society is in a state of serious struggle. Put some of the simple beauty of nature back in your life. We have lost touch with simplicity in our rush for "progress."

[] [] [] [] [] []

A **summary** on the **principles of wellness** would not be complete without listing these highlights that should be top priority in your quest for well being.

* *The more you stick to* **supplements that contain NATURAL WHOLE FOODS,** *the more likely you are to achieve the results you desire. Any multiple vitamin and mineral supplement should contain micronutrients from whole foods, and herbs in the formula.*

* Live in **conformity with the body's circadian rhythm**. Make every effort to have a bowel elimination, and eat light before noon; and do not eat a heavy meal after 8 PM. Get more than one half of your night's sleep before 4 AM.

* **Raw and unprocessed foods** best provide the nutrients your body needs to perform its many functions. Our low intake of **essential fatty acids** that are deficient in processed food, is a major contributing factor in many common diseases. Eat *alive* foods like whole grains, cold-pressed oils, raw nuts and seeds.

* **Eliminate red meat and dairy products**; or consume in small amounts for *occasional* social situations. *Animal products should be hormone and antibiotic free.* When eating out, order fish or seafood.

* When **chlorine** combines with the natural organic matter in the water, volatile pollutants are formed (like chloroform) that can cause disease. An inexpensive **shower filter** can protect the skin from the toxins

created by chlorinated water. **Drinking water should be filtered regardless of the source.** Filtered water should also eliminate **Fluoride.** Fluoride is more poisonous than lead, and just slightly less poisonous than arsenic. While no one will die from one glass of fluoridated water, just as no one will die from smoking one cigarette, it is the long-term chronic effects of daily continuous exposure to fluoridated water and products, that takes its toll in human health. Collectively you can get Fluoride from drinking water, treatments at the dentists, toothpaste, mouthwash, fluoride drops, and some food preparation.

* **Fitness** can be gained or lost in a 28-day period. Any daily exercise must include impact to the bottom of the feet to move the lymphatic system.

* *Test your **urine and saliva pH** once a month for the rest of your life!* Mark it on your calendar; this is too important to forget!!! If your pH is abnormal, so is your digestion, and your ability to deal with stress.

* *Test your **temperature** once a month lifetime.* If it is below 98.4 orally, refer to the thyroid section in the Internal Energy chapter. *This is critical health evaluation, because it goes to the very basis of your body's ability to utilize nutrients for fuel and energy.*

* **Minerals** are easily lost in the typical American diet. Minerals are the catalysts in the chemical reactions that go on in the body every day. Minerals like calcium, magnesium, potassium, and sodium are "electrolytes" that transmit electrical nerve impulses. Unprocessed seasalt is like a tonic for electrolyte balance.

* **Supplementing Q10** provides the raw material needed to activate intracellular energy. Q10 is produced in the liver. However, pH imbalance, poor digestion, and a

liver stressed from modern day abuse reduces the production of this critical nutrient. Get rid of some toxic wastes that are hard on the liver, with a *two to three times yearly* general cleansing program.

* **Supplementing methylsulfonylmethane (MSM)** which is a key nutritional ingredient available in all plant and animal life. It is essential to a healthy diet. Even though it is found in almost every fresh food of any origin, it is extremely volatile. MSM is rapidly lost when food is processed, or consumed anytime later than "just picked." **ALMOST ANY SYMPTOM OF THE BODY CAN BENEFIT FROM MSM SUPPLEMENTATION.** MSM is safe at any beneficial dose, with no known toxic levels. Maintenance may produce results at 1000 milligrams two times a day. Acute conditions may do better at 4000 milligrams three times a day, then reduce as symptoms improve.

* The body's immune system is too often stretched to the breaking point. Supplements with **antioxidants** like Vitamins A, C, E, Zinc, Selenium, Grape Seed Extract, Green Tea Extract, Glutamine, and Lipoic Acid (a universal antioxidant), help fight off the damage produced by modern day living. Check out products for immune system support.

* Too often people concentrate on the symptom and not on the bottom line cause. The **pituitary** is the forgotten gland in the quest for health. It supports the immune system, influences the growth of skin, bones, muscles and organs throughout the body. Sleep, energy, and elevated moods are appreciated benefits. Good digestion, stress management, B vitamins, anti-oxidants, herb vitex available in health food stores, exercise, and massaging the bottom inner side of the big toe, all are supports for pituitary function.

*   Be more conscious of your rights as a **nonsmoker**. If you are a smoker consider these "quit smoking" techniques:

    -   Do a thorough self analysis, and determine what lost pleasure you have experienced, that made you substitute what you consider to be a "pleasurable" alternative.

    -   Understand that smoking has become a substitute "friend." Do you really want such a destructive "friend." Would you expect a "friend" to negatively affect you?

    -   Find a healthier "friend" to support you until you release the past, and get on with the challenge of developing your life's goals ... and building your self-esteem!

    -   Get out of the "I" and into "we" thinking. That will automatically make you more considerate about destructive second hand smoke, or the way you smell. This form of compassionate growth will give "you" unlimited rewards.

    -   Evaluate your dietary choices, and follow the "laws" of wellness to eliminate stress that encourages addictions.

    -   Eliminate all fruit, fruit juices, natural and refine sugars until your sugar cravings subside.

    -   Some people have been successful reducing the number of cigarettes daily. For example, if you smoked a pack a day, each day put one less in a separate pack, and spread the allowed number out over the day. This really works if you are honest about the reduction.

- Every day say multiple affirmations that you make healthy choices for your well-being. Do not put a negative in your affirmation like "I do not smoke." Affirmations should always be positive.

* Be aware that **birth control pills** can produce an energetic defiance of glandular health. Instead of the glands being capable of balance, they go into chaos from blockage in the distribution centers for glandular energy. Do not mess with Mother Nature! There are safer options for birth control, and options for other reasons birth control pills are prescribed.

* Nutrients that are excellent to support male **prostate health** include Lycopene and Saw palmetto.

* Examples of foods like soybeans and canola oil are only the tip of the iceberg as genetically engineered foods becomes a controversial health issue. Look for non GMO labeled foods, as public alarm for his potential health concern will require foods to be labeled informatively.

* Start every day, first thing in the morning with a *positive attitude,* and your *game plan.* You should now be ready to work on your *life wish. It takes both enthusiasm and action to make something happen!* **KEEP FOCUSED!!! DO NOT LOSE YOUR PERSONAL POWER!!!**

"IF WE DID ALL THE THINGS WE ARE CAPABLE OF DOING, WE WOULD LITERALLY ASTONISH OURSELVES."

- Thomas Edison

MAKE THE START OF EACH DAY SPECIAL!

"I EXPECT TO PASS THROUGH THIS WORLD BUT ONCE. ANY GOOD THEREFORE THAT I CAN DO, OR ANY KINDNESS OR ABILITIES THAT I CAN SHOW TO ANY FELLOW CREATURE, LET ME DO IT NOW. LET ME NOT DEFER OR NEGLECT IT, FOR I SHALL NOT PASS THIS WAY AGAIN."

- William Penn

*   Besides the recommendations for physical health, you need to **connect with your spiritual beliefs**, and let the direction you get from your Creator guide you to bring out your strengths, and *turn your lights on*. If your positive thoughts are creative, progressive, innovative, or improvement thoughts, **LISTEN TO THEM!!!** Allow yourself to *open up* ... A HIGHER POWER MAY BE TALKING TO YOU! *I love this refrain from the hymn "Here I Am Lord" by Shute and Young:*

> *Here I am, Lord,*
> *Is it I, Lord?*
> *I have heard you calling in the night.*
> *I will go, Lord, if you lead me,*
> *I will hold your people in my heart.*

Webster's dictionary describes spiritual as "of the spirit or the soul, as distinguished from the body of material matters." There is a sensitivity to Spirituality that removes it from the collection of human experiences, and places it on the outside of our existence. Spirituality is like a butterfly passing through our limited vision. We reach for it, and it too often seems to lie just beyond our grasp. In special moments we may feel Spirituality moving within us as we feel calm, gentle and balanced. The meaning of life that expresses love and kindness seems natural. But this

287

feeling is, for too many of us, fleeting. We return to a world of "material concerns." We return to "the real world, and the efforts needed to survive." We too often, or too late, fail to understand that the peace felt within us would make dealing with any stressful effort easier.

... there came to me, I cannot tell whence, a most powerful sweetness that had never come to me before. It was not religious, like the goodness of a text heard at a preaching. It was beyond that.

- Mary Webb - British Poet

Spirituality can best be described as a way of life, and refers to our hopes and dreams; our patterns of thought, emotions, feelings and behaviors. Spirituality is not something we bring out for special occasions like clothing, but what we wear in our heart and mind everyday. That is where boundaries are established that express our morals, our values, the core of our being, and who we are. A spiritual person has qualities that include serenity and confidence. We feel comfortable with people who have strong boundaries, and are not judgmental.

"Let no one ever come to you without leaving better and happier. Be the living expression of kindness in your face, kindness in your eyes, and kindness in your smile."

- Mother Teresa

One story I heard was about a man who was asked what Spirituality meant to him. Eager to make an impression of his own intelligence, he gave a huge, complex detailed explanation that went on for most of lunch. After describing every theory he had ever studied or heard about, he asked what Spirituality meant to others. His lunch companion looked at him gently, took a sip of water and said, "Spirituality is kindness."

288

"Practice being kind rather than right."

- Wayne Dyer

Being human we have choices other species do not have. Life is a classroom where we are all given lessons to learn. The subject of Spirituality cannot be adequately covered in this short section. My hope is that these few words act as a flag, rising up in you feelings that will encourage you to learn and grow on all levels of spiritual, mental, emotional, and physical.

[] [] [] [] [] []

It is sensible to practice the *PRINCIPLES OF HEALTH*, and prevent disease rather than to treat all the individual symptoms. Since the body is an interrelated system, it is important to treat *THE WHOLE BODY AT ONE TIME*, and not just a single area of concern. Even some health-oriented books support separate body areas by dealing with individual subjects, like nutrition in one book, elimination in another, exercise in another, and personal development in still another. THE BODY SHOULD BE TREATED AS A UNIT ... SIMPLY, AND WITH RECOMMENDATIONS THAT ARE BACK-TO-BASICS. *THE POWER TO HEAL* has attempted to teach you the importance of the interrelation between all levels of spiritual, mental, emotional, and physical!

"It is supposed to be a professional secret, but I'll tell you anyway. We doctors do nothing. We only help encourage the doctor within.

- Dr. Albert Schweitzer

Relationships, careers, and social pressures, are being handled by people with chronic health problems. Self pacification with social temptations is easy in a mentally and physically exhausted body. **We must look at issues that**

289

formulate our cellular ability to have a positive or negative attitude. Look at our intake of social and prescription drugs. **Look at** electromagnetic polluted frequencies in our industrialized world. **Look at** our totally chemical society since World War II. **Look at** too many positive and too few negative ions from our "new and improved" world. **Look at** a society so unknowledgeable about healthy choices that being health oriented is a joke. **Look at** children who admire bullies and fanatics, instead of spiritual leaders or health teachers. **Look at** the decline in family unity. No one seems to know how to stop societies runaway train. **There has never been a greater need for health recommendation that "simply" work!**

Wellness does not have to be a difficult subject. Learn how to deal with tension and stress through **positive thinking.** Eat food that is *capable* of providing high quality **nutrition.** Consume chemical and parasite free **water.** Be conscious of good **digestion** principles. Help your body **eliminate waste** products at a speed that allows cells to function at peak performance. **Exercise** to *ENJOY LIFE* and promote a healthy circulatory and lymphatic system. Protect yourself from modern day **polluted frequencies.** This all adds up to *COMMON SENSE! DO NOT GET LOST IN DETAILS.* No given day is a test of all your knowledge perfectly implemented. Relax ... enjoy your learning experience. Take *pride* in learning how to take responsibility for your health. **Make sensible choices! Take care of your body ... and your body will take care of you.**

We spend money on health insurance, which is not the treatment of health, but of disease. **The "laws" of wellness in this book are "health insurance."** Researching alternative therapies has given me an inside look at what really goes on in this society, with our medical approach to the treatment of disease. We have made life saving advance in some areas, but have mistake some "advances" as an improvement on the "laws" of wellness. I hope this book will renew your faith in the healing power of the principles that allow the body to heal itself.

❑ ❑ ❑ ❑ ❑ ❑

TO MAINTAIN THE LEVEL OF WELLNESS THAT ALLOWS YOU TO ENJOY LIFE TO THE FULLEST, EXPAND YOUR KNOWLEDGE ON:

POSITIVE THINKING

NUTRITION

DIGESTION

ELIMINATION

EXERCISE

USING THE FOLLOWING PRINCIPLES ON A REGULAR BASIS:

ROTATION

MODERATION

BALANCE

COMMON SENSE

UNDERSTANDING THE FOLLOWING "LAWS" OF WELLNESS:

WATER

TRACE MINERALS

ESSENTIAL FATTY ACIDS

pH BALANCE

CONTROL OF CANDIDA YEAST AND PARASITES

ELIMINATION

DAILY LYMPHATIC AND CARDIOVASCULAR EXERCISE, MUSCLE TONE, AND OXYGEN

STRESS MANAGEMENT

The trigger that can release a latent cancer can be a personal misfortune or profound frustration that results in a despair about ever achieving real personal happiness. A person's **attitude** toward life helps determine the stress to the immune system.

UNDERSTANDING THAT BODY STRESS CAN ALSO COME FROM:

ROOT CANALS THAT CAN LEAK BACTERIA EVEN THOUGH THEY ARE NOT INFECTED, AND OLD MERCURY FILLINGS.

"I now rank root canals right behind mercury amalgam fillings as a cause of ill health, and with an estimated 60 million root canals performed in 1998, you can appreciate the scope of the problem."

- Whole Body Dentistry by Mark A. Breiner, DDS

EXPOSURE TO ELECTROMAGNETIC POLLUTED FREQUENCIES FROM OUR INDUSTRIALIZED SOCIETY

FEMALE HORMONAL IMBALANCES – This society is still following standards set by the medical profession. The belief is that their concentration of estrogen replacement must then be right. A growing

292

number of women upset with the established order of things, have studied recognized work on progesterone by Dr. John Lee, M.D. (in Resource References). There are safer, natural alternatives to synthetic hormone replacement therapy that actually PROTECT female health, and not put you at risk for cancer, heart disease, osteoporosis and a host of other illnesses. Learning the risks of synthetic hormones versus the benefits of natural hormones could save your life! Do not be sold a bill of goods that only helps the drug companies.

Knowledge is power in preventing breast cancer. Besides following the "laws" of wellness in this book, women should never wear underwires, and should always wear bras that do not feel tight. You can enlarge any bra with an extender to improve lymphatic flow that drains toxic wastes from the breast. A diet high in "soy everything" is not recommended because the phytoestrogens can disrupt endocrine function. Plastic in microwaves converts to phytoestrogens, so "technologically advance" continues to bring surprises. Digital Infrared Thermography is a safe screening technique that is safer and more accurate than mammograms.

ALLERGIC REACTIONS TO MICROSCOPIC BED MITES. REMEMBER TO …

- *shower every night before going to bed, with a good vigorous skin brushing.*

- *wash you sheets weekly.*

- *wash your mattress pad monthly.*

- *vacuum your bed monthly.*

- *consider covering your mattress and pillows with mite free barrier cloth products – check Resources References.*

TOXICITY FROM INGESTED OR EXPOSURE TO POISONS LIKE MERCURY, CHLORINE, AND FLUORIDE.

"The greatest advances in medicine have not been the discovery of new technology ... but in prevention."

- Health Financial Management Journal June 1990

I hope by now The power To Heal has your attention. **You must first understand all the body needs, as a whole unit.** Without that overview, you might be disappointed at the result of your effort. You may now want to increase your knowledge with a book dedicated to a particular subject you want to understand better. *There is no limit when you challenge your desire to learn.*

[] [] [] [] [] []

Discussion on the fundamentals of health would not be complete without some reference to THE MEANING OF LIFE. The most primal and basic human need is the need for meaning. Satisfy the meaning of existence for you, and you will make better choices to protect the new found quality of life. *Instead of discussing symptoms and disease in the doctor's office, you will be concentrating on the promotion of wellness in your home!* The meaning of your life is a very private matter, and so should be your right to search in your own way. **Searching for your personal power is a joyful lifetime adventure!**

294

Power is spelled COMMITMENT, and that means commitment to:

- personal growth

- personal contribution of mankind.

**IMPROVED HEALTH WILL FOLLOW
AS SURELY AS DAY FOLLOWS NIGHT!**

[] [] [] [] [] []

So, dear reader, we have reached the end of a pleasant journey together. You have increased your health knowledge about prevention of disease since you first opened this book. You now understand that the body functions through energy such as:

- *Energy from positive mental thoughts and emotional feelings*

- *Energy the body needs to function, instead of protecting you from negative polluted frequencies.*

- *Synergistic energy from supplements that contain natural food and herb sources, and not drug look-a-likes that lacks synergy to work together.*

- *Energy from exercise.*

- *Energy from healthy water.*

- *Energy from unprocessed foods.*

- *Energy from color therapy (articles and filters can be obtained from Second Opinion newsletters by Robert Jay Rowen, MD. Refer to Resource References)*

295

As you close the back cover, you will open a door to the rest of your life. THE POWER TO HEAL *will* always be on your library shelf, to freshen your memory, or just to remind you that assuming self-responsibility for your health is exciting and rewarding. You can now develop your own self-confidence, dedication to your well being, and an enthusiasm for life that will make daily decisions easier. Through your **health metamorphosis** you will discover challenges and make plans that will give new meaning to your life. I congratulate you on completing this book ... you are worth it!

"EDUCATION IS NOT PREPARATION FOR LIFE. EDUCATION IS LIFE ITSELF."

- John Dewey

I saw a page of stickers that include words like Good Job, Hooray, Terrific, Bravo, Wonderful, Excellent, Great, You're Special, Super, WOW, Awesome, Brilliant, and You Rule. **BECAUSE YOU ARE TAKING RESPONSIBILITY FOR YOUR WELLNESS... YOU GET THEM ALL!!!**

HAVE A GREAT LIFE!!!

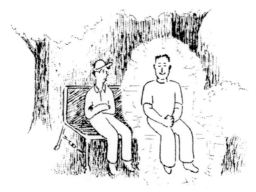

I take it you're using those
ALTERNATIVE MEDICINES again !?

RESOURCE REFERENCES

The following references are based on current availability. Books frequently go out of print or have the title changed on reprints, phone numbers and addresses may change. If you cannot find a book, a bookstore can help you learn the current status. If you need assistance with resource references, my ˙ website is kept current: www.thehealingpower.com.

THE FOLLOWING BOOKS ARE **RESOURCE REFERENCES:**

* **Alternative Medicine - The Definitive Guide -** compiled by the Burton Goldberg Group - 1998 - Future Medicine Publishing, Inc., 5009 Pacific Hwy. E, Suite 6, Fife, WA 98424.

* **Apple Cider Vinegar, Miracle Health System -** by Paul and Patricia Bragg - c.1998 - Health Science, Box 7, Santa Barbara, CA 93102; 1-800-446-1990; www.bragg.com.

* **Dr. Whitaker's Guide To Natural Healing -** Julian Whitaker, M.D. -1996 - Prima Publishing, P.O. Box 1260BK, Rocklin, CA 95677; 1-916-632-4440.

* **Earl Mindell's Secret Remedies** – Earl Mindell, R.Ph., Ph.D. – 1997 Simon & Schuster, Fireside Books, Rockefeller Center, 1230 Ave. of the Americas, New York, NY 10020.

* **Earl Mindell's Soy Miracle** – Earl Mindell, R.Ph., Ph.D. – 1995 – Simon & Schuster, Fireside Books, Rockefeller Center, 1230 Ave. of the Americas, New York, NY 10020.

* **Earl Mindell's Vitamin Bible** – Earl Mindell, R.Ph., Ph.D. – 1985, 1991, 1998 – Warner Books, 666 Fifth Ave., New York, NY 10103.

* **Prescription Alternatives** – Earl Mindell, R.Ph., Ph.D & Virginia Hopkins, M.A., 2nd Edition 1989, Kents Publishing, Inc., 27 Pine St., Box 876, New Canaan, CT 06840-0876.

* **The Biochemic Handbook: How to get Well and Keep Fit with Biochemic Tissue Salts,** J.B. Chapman M.D./Edward L Perry M.D., Formur International.

* **Cancer Cover-up** by Kathleen Deoul can be ordered at www.cassandrabooks.com. A highly recommended book filled with documented information the medical profession does not want you to know.

* **The Chemistry of Man** - Bernard Jensen, Ph.D. - 1983 – Bernard Jensen Enterprises, 24360 Old Wagon Road, Escondido, CA 92027.

* **The Cure For All Diseases** - Hulda Regehr Clark, Ph.D., N.D. – 1995 Promotion Publishing, 3368F Governor Drive, Suite 144, San Diego, CA 92122. Also, **The Cure For all Cancers.**

* **The Golden Seven Plus One (Conquer Disease with Eight Keys to Health, Beauty, and Peace)** - C. Samuel West, D.N., N.D. - 1981 -Samuel Publishing Co., P.O. Box 1051, Orem, UT 84059; 1-800-975-0123.

* **Silver Dental Filling: The Toxic Time Bomb,** Sam Ziff – 1985 – Aurora Press, 205 3rd Ave., 2A, NewYork, NY 10003.

* **Toxic Metal Syndrome – How Much Metal Poisonings Can Affect Your Brain** – Dr. H. Richard

Casdorph, Dr. Morton Walker – 1995 Avery Publishing Group, Garden City Park, NY.

* **The Yeast Connection** - William G. Crook, M.D. - 1983 – Professional Books, P.O. Box 3246, Jackson, TN 38303.

* **What Your Doctor May *Not* Tell You About Premenopause** and also **What Your Doctor May *Not* Tell You About Menopause** – John R. Lee, M.D. – 1999 – Warner Books, Inc., 1271 Avenue of the Americas, New York, NY 10020

* **Whole Body Dentistry – Discover the Missing Piece to Better Health** – Mark A. Breiner, DDS, Robert C. Atkins, M.D. (Introduction) – 1999 - Quantum Health Press, LLC P.O. Box 1637, Fairfield, CT 06432, 1-800-BOOKLOG.

* **Your Body's Many Cries For Water** - F. Batmanghelidj, M.D. – 1995 - Global Health Solutions, 2146 Kings Garden Way, Falls Church, VA 22043; 1-703-848-2333.

[] [] [] [] [] []

*THE FOLLOWING BOOKS ARE **EXCELLENT** ADDITIONS TO YOUR WELLNESS LIBRARY. ANY BOOKSTORE CAN ORDER FOR YOU, OR CHECK CURRENT AVAILABILITY:*

* **Acid & Alkaline** - Herman Aihara - 1986 - George Ohsawa Macrobiotic Foundation, 1511 Robinson Street, Oroville, CA 95965.

* **Alkalize or Die** - Theodore A. Baroody, N.D., D.C., Ph.D. Nutrition, C.N.C. - 1991 - Eclectic Press, 205 Pigeon Street, Waynesville, NC 28786; 1-800-566-1522.

* **The Bach Flower Remedies** – Incorporating **Heal Thyself, The Twelve Healers, The Bach Remedies Repertory,** Edward Bach and F. J. Wheeler, 1997 – Keats Publishing, Inc., 27 Pine Street (Box 876), New Canaan, CN 06840.

* **Bach Flower Therapy, Theory and Practice** – Mechthild Scheffer – 1988 – Healing Arts Press, One Park Street, Rochester, VT 05767.

* **Dr. Abravanel's Body Type Diet and Lifetime Nutrition Plan** – Eliot D. Abravanel, M.D. - 1999 - Bantam Books, Inc., New York, NY 10103.

* **3 - Day Cleanse, Mucusless Diet** - John Christopher – Christopher Publications, 1-800-372-8255.

* **Everybody's Guide to Homeopathic Medicines** – Stephen Cummings, F.N.P., Dana Ullman, M.P.H. – 1997 – Jeremy P. Tarcher, Inc., 9110 Sunset Blvd.,Los Angeles, CA 90069.

* **Happiness Is A Serious Problem, A Human Nature Repair Manuel** – Dennis Prager – Harper Collins, 1-800-242-7737.

* **How to Survive the Loss of a Love** - Melba Colgrove, Ph.D., Harold H. Bloomfield, M.D., Peter McWilliams - 1993 - Bantam Books, New York.

* **If It's Going To Be, It's Up To Me** – Robert H. Schuller – 1997 – Harper Collins; 1-800-9POWER9. Powerful spiritual guidance.

* **Milk – The Deadly Poison** – Robert Cohen – 1997 – Argus Publishing, Inc., 301 Sylvan Ave., Englewood Cliffs, NJ 07632.

302

* **Pocket Manual of Homeopathic Materia Medica and Repertory** –William Boericke, M.D. - 1982 - Boericke & Runyon, Philadelphia, PA (Source for Homeopathic Remedy information).

* **Reinventing _Your_ Church** – Brian D. McLaren – may be ordered through bookstores, or publisher, Zondervan Publishing House, Grand Rapids, Michigan 49530, 1-616-698-6900.

* **Sea Salt's Hidden Powers** – The Grain and Salt Society, 273 Fairway Dr., Asheville, NC 28805, 1-800-867-7258.

* **The Essiac Report: Canada's Remarkable Unknown Cancer Remedy** - Richard Thomas - 1994 - The Alternative Treatment Information Network, 1244 Ozeta Terrace, Los Angeles, CA 90069; 1-310-278-6611.

* **The Herb Book** - John Lust, N.D., D.B.M. - 1983 - Bantam Books, Inc., New York, NY 10103.

* **The New Herb Bible** – Earl Mindell, R.Ph., Ph.D. – 1999 – Simon & Schuster, Rockefeller Center, 1230 Ave. of the Americas, New York, NY 10020.

* **The New Possibility Thinkers Bible** - Robert H. Schuller and Paul David Dunn - 1996 - Thomas Nelson Publishers; 1-800-976-9379.

[] [] [] [] []

RECOMMENDED SPEAKERS, VIDEOS, TAPES, SPIRITUAL LEADERS AND HOLISTIC SOURCE INFORMATION:

* **"Alternatives" newsletter** by Dr. David Williams contains information for the health-conscious individual. To order call 1-800-219-8591

* **Center for Natural Medicine**, Martin Milner M.D., 1330 S.E. 39 th Avenue, Portland, Oregon 97214; 1-503-232-1100; Fax 1-503-232-7751; drmilner@hotmail.com.

* **"Health & Healing" newsletter** by Julian Whitaker, M.D. is your definitive guide to alternative health and anti-aging medicine. To order call 1-800-539-8219.

* **www.oxytherapy.com** for information on oxygen spa therapy.

* **"Second Opinion"** by Robert Jay Rowen, M.D., P.O. Box 467939, Atlanta, Georgia, 31146-7939, 1-800-728-2288. Source for information on therapeutic use of color.

* **SPEAKER AGENCIES:**

  Thom Lisk Professional Speakers Group, 1-800-705-0079; www.terrificspeakers.com.

* **INSPIRATIONAL SPEAKERS:**

* **Ellen Kreidman, Ph.D.,** Personal relationship audio tapes; www.lightyourfire.com.

* **Joyce Meyer Ministries** – Spiritual approaches to personal growth; 1-800-707-7877; television, videos, tapes, and books; www.jmministries.org.

304

*   **Ed Young** – Spiritual approach to personal growth; 1-800-301-9255; television, videos, tapes, and books; www.winningwalk.org.

*   **Robert Schuller** – Possibility Thinking Spirituality, 1-800-9POWER9; television, videos, tapes, and books; call for catalog; www.crystalcathedral.org.

*   **James Kennedy** – Coral Ridge Ministries, 1-800-892-9855; television, videos, tapes, and books; www.coralridge.org.

*   **Arthur Caliandro** – home church replacement for Norman Vincent Peale. Excellent spiritual leader and teacher of positive development. For more information call 1-800-626-2724, or www.marblevision.org.

*   **Edgar Cayce Books and Videos for Personal Growth** - Call 1-800-723-1112 to request a catalog; www.edgarcayce.org.

*   **John Hagee Ministries**, television, videos, tapes, and book.1-800-854-9899. WWW.jhm.org.

*   **Joel Osteen**, Pastor Lakewood Church, Houston, Texas, television, videos, tapes, 1-800-828-5228.

CATALOGS:

Janice's Natural Comfort Collection -Natural clothing and bedding.1-800-526-4237.
www.janices.com.

The Vermont Country Store—Natural and hard to find items. 1-802-362-8470.
www.vermontcountrystore.com

Needs—Nutrition, ecological, and environment products.1-800-634-1380.
www.needs.com

A GUIDE TO PRODUCT AVAILABILITY:

NOTE: Health Expos are exciting ways to find out the newest in health and fitness products. Check your local newspaper, and attend any large or small health shows in your area! That is the best way to keep up on current health trends, new products, and new supplements. If you cannot attend health expos, check your health food store for magazine or newsletter information, or books that will keep you current. There are many professionals advertising health newsletters. You will find your favorite in your quest for wellness. You can get resource information on my website www.thehealingpower.com.

INDEX

ABOUT THE AUTHOR

THE PERSONAL HEALTH SUCCESS STORY:

For 20 years, Dori was chronically ill, and struggling with poor health on all levels of mental, emotional, and physical. She became so ill she was often bed-ridden, and the quality of life was gone. Life itself became a challenge in survival. Finally, she found doctors who treated the CAUSE of illness instead of just the symptoms. She learned the "laws" of wellness, and experienced an incredible metamorphosis. The cocoon of a sickly body became a healthy, vital person. Now at 68, people meeting her for the first time marvel at her vitality, energy and enthusiasm. People who knew her during her many years of illness are amazed at her improved health.

THE PROFESSIONAL:

Dori has been a leader in the health field for 47 years. Past career work that has contributed to her holistic view of wellness includes two prevention oriented health clinics for 12 years, a rehabilitation nurse for two years, three years of personal development seminars, and a psychiatric nurse for 6 years. That background, her Naturopathic Doctor diploma, and eight years as a Naturopathic practitioner gives her insight into all aspects of wellness and stress management.

THE SPEAKER:

Dori is a trained professional in public speaking through National Speakers Association, and delivers speeches, seminars, and courses on stress management, and self-responsibility in health care. She is a one-stop source of information on all levels of spiritual, mental, emotional, and physical. Her credits include radio and television appearances.

THE AUTHOR:

Dori's first book FOUNTAIN OF HEALTH AND FITNESS and the 1st edition of her second book HEALTH METAMORPHOSIS is out of print. She is still distributing the 2nd edition of HEALTH METAMORPHOSIS. Twenty years of holistic research is culminated in her latest book, THE POWER TO HEAL. She has written a regular health article for a newspaper for 6 years. She plans to submit more articles to educational health resources. Her future writing plans include focusing on the health of children and young adults. That is the age group that desperately needs health education.

HOW TO ORDER "THE POWER TO HEAL"

TO ORDER ADDITIONAL COPIES CALL 1ST BOOKS LIBRARY 1-888-280-7715.

TO ORDER 100 COPIES OR MORE FOR DISCOUNT, CALL 1ST BOOKS LIBRARY 1-888-519-5121 Extension 219, or FAX 1-812-339-6554. Allow three to four weeks for delivery.

Printed in the United States
704600003B